It Could Happen
to You or a Loved One

(C) Jim Knox, a 55-year-old air traffic controller outside Seattle, sat in a darkened room with two other controllers, watching lights move across the radar screen. Dick Bobb, the traffic manager on duty and one of Jim's oldest friends, noticed Jim slumped forward with his head resting on his control board as he made his tour of the room.

"Traffic that slow, Jimmy?" Dick quipped. To his alarm, Jim did not respond. "Jimmy, can you hear me?" he shouted. Still, there was no response.

Supervisor Ed Gass came over to Jim, lifted his head, and realized that he was unconscious. He told Dick Bobb, "I think Jimmy's had a heart attack." Ed checked Jim for a pulse, and wasn't able to find one. . . .

WOULD YOU KNOW WHAT
EMERGENCY ACTION TO TAKE?

*(See the chapter "Heart Attack
and Cardiac Arrest")*

D0910878

THE
RESCUE
911™

FAMILY
FIRST AID &
EMERGENCY
CARE BOOK

JULIE MOTZ

POCKET BOOKS
New York   London   Toronto   Sydney   Tokyo   Singapore

The author of this book is not a physician. The rescue and medical practices presented in this book are specific to the circumstances. Every medical emergency is different and recommended procedures may vary accordingly. In the event of a medical or health emergency, you should promptly contact a local emergency service and/or a trained health professional. The author and publisher disclaim any liability arising directly or indirectly as a result of the information, practices or advice presented in this book.

An *Original* Publication of POCKET BOOKS

POCKET BOOKS, a division of Simon & Schuster Inc.
1230 Avenue of the Americas, New York, NY 10020

ISBN: 0-671-52514-X

First Pocket Books printing May 1996

10 9 8 7 6 5 4 3 2 1

POCKET and colophon are registered trademarks of Simon & Schuster Inc.

Text design by Stanley S. Drate, Folio Graphics Co. Inc.

Printed in the U.S.A.

To my father, Lloyd Motz

I would like to thank Jim Milio from "Rescue 911," my agent Janis Vallely, my editor Emily Bestler, and her associate Amelia Sheldon for all of their help.

Emergency Telephone Numbers

In most areas of the country, "9-1-1" is the number to call to put you in touch with emergency medical personnel. To find your local emergency number, look inside the cover of your phone book or call your local hospital. When you call the emergency number, be prepared to give your address and to describe calmly, as completely as possible, what the situation is, including the time of onset of the problem.

If there is no central coordinating emergency number for your area, call the fire department, the police department, or the hospital emergency department, as needed. If you cannot find these numbers, dial "0" (zero) and ask the operator for help.

All local emergency numbers should be posted by each phone in your home and children should be taught how to call in an emergency.

Local emergency phone: _____

Family physician: _____

Pediatrician: _____

Poison control center: _____

Hospital emergency department: _____

Fire: _____

Police: _____

Local pharmacy: _____

24-hour pharmacy: _____

Gas company: _____

Electric company: _____

Relative or neighbor: _____

Mother's phone at work: _____

Father's phone at work: _____

Emergency First-Aid Supplies

It is a good idea to keep an emergency first-aid kit in an accessible, dry place in your home and to make certain that all family members know where it is. Replace used supplies regularly. The kit should include:

- Sterile gauze pads (dressings), 2 and 4 inches square, to place over wounds
- Roll of gauze bandage 3 inches wide to hold dressings in place
- Triangular bandages for making arm slings and holding dressings in place
- Adhesive bandages in various sizes
- Roll of 1-inch adhesive tape
- 3-inch elastic bandage for wrapping sprained ankles and wrists
- Blunt-ended scissors
- Safety pins
- Roll of absorbent cotton to use as padding with splints
- Antiseptic wipes
- Tweezers
- Cotton swabs
- Ice bag or chemical ice pack

- Disposable gloves, such as surgical or examination gloves
- Syrup of ipecac
- Bar of plain soap
- Flashlight, with extra batteries in a separate bag

Contents

Foreword

Many wonderful surprises have come from producing "Rescue 911," but none so gratifying as having more than 300 lives saved because of the show. Viewers, including very young children, watched episodes of "Rescue 911" and later, when an emergency struck, remembered what they saw and did what was needed to save a life. This is an amazing tribute to the positive power of television.

This book will help readers learn about emergencies and how to handle them, but more importantly, it tells how to prevent needless injuries from occurring in the first place by being aware and being prepared.

The faster victims receive proper help, the more likely their survival. The producers of "Rescue 911" recommend that everyone, including children, take a cardiopulmonary resuscitation class, available through the American Red Cross and the American Heart Association.

May you and your family enjoy a very safe life!

Jim Milio
Producer/Director
"Rescue 911"
Hollywood, California

Introduction

It has become a common complaint that we are a country that has lost its heroes. Every year, though, thousands of Americans face life-and-death situations in their own homes and deal with them calmly, courageously, and heroically. And every day, all across the country, emergency medical technicians, many of them summoned to the scene of an accident or other emergency through the 9-1-1 rescue system, save lives and prevent disasters.

"Rescue 911" is a program that celebrates the heroism of ordinary people who find themselves unexpectedly dealing with situations where death or serious injury seems imminent. It also educates the public about how to respond to emergencies and keep them from becoming tragedies.

Early in 1989, Kim LeMasters, then president of CBS Entertainment, was driving to work when he heard a story on the radio about a very dramatic rescue, initiated by a call to 9-1-1. He was convinced that this kind of material could make exciting television, and he called Norman Powell, head of in-house production at the network, to discuss it.

Powell called documentary producer Arnold Sha-
piro, who developed three pilots for CBS with co-
producer Jean O'Neill. After the first two shows
were aired that spring, CBS believed it had a winner
and decided to turn it into a series. Since then, over
170 "Rescue 911" episodes have been aired.

Every week, the producers of the program choose
from among 500 to 1,000 possible stories. They
come from phone calls and letters from viewers,
newspaper clips, computer networks, and the work
of the research staff, who are in touch with police
departments, fire departments, hospital emergency
departments, and 9-1-1 centers around the country.
To qualify for production, the stories must be inter-
esting, unusual, medically accurate, and not show
anyone doing anything dangerous or inadvisable,
such as a nonprofessional running into a burning
building (which usually results in death). Finally,
in the vast majority of cases, they must contain a
definitive safety lesson. "We don't just want to take
people on a white-knuckle roller-coaster ride," says
the producer/director for the show, Jim Milio.

Although some people have complained that the
show doesn't present any failures ("We leave that
to the tabloid shows and the evening news," Milio
says. "Basically, we want to show that the system
can and does work"), the response from both the
public and emergency professionals has been over-
whelmingly positive. Paramedics and 9-1-1 dispatchers, in particular, are grateful that their jobs
are so well explained. The show has brought to the
public's awareness the fact that paramedics don't
just transport people to hospitals. They are medically trained and frequently give treatment at the

scene of the emergency that saves lives. Similarly, it has allowed people to understand why phone dispatchers ask all the questions they do, and what they do with the information.

In many cases, people have written to the show's producers to tell them that they had been uncertain about what they wanted to do professionally, but that watching the show convinced them to become an emergency professional. "We also get a lot of letters from people who tell us that the show restores their faith in humanity by letting them see that there are a lot of selfless people who will go that extra mile, and even risk their lives for somebody else," Milio says. "And we know that many people take actions they normally wouldn't have because of the show. They write to us—like the woman who sent us the frayed extension cord she found burning the back of her dresser when she checked it after seeing a program about the dangers of fire started by old extension cords."

So far as is possible, the program tries to have real people playing themselves, unless it's too dangerous or too emotionally upsetting for them to relive the situation. When they do, it's usually enjoyable, and often cathartic. Sometimes, just the interviewing done by the director can result in a healing experience for the people involved. Jim Milio explains:

"When people go through a really bad trauma—a life-or-death situation—many times, they don't talk about it when it's over, not even with their family or their loved ones—they just bottle it up. When our directors show up, they ask them really intimate things, like, 'What did you feel like when you saw your husband lying there, virtually dead? Did you imagine life without him? Did you think he was going to make it?' These are questions that in many cases no one has ever asked them—stuff they've never said to anybody. And then we find that after we've interviewed the family, they start talking to one another about it. 'What did you say?' 'Well, I said this . . .' 'You felt that way? I didn't know that.' And all of a sudden, they're talking about a really significant incident in their lives that they've never discussed before. In many cases, this helps relieve the guilt or shame of someone who feels that his or her neglect caused the accident."

The idea of a universal emergency number originated in Great Britain (where 999 was chosen as the number), and was activated there in 1937. The first 9-1-1 service on this continent was implemented in 1968 in Nome, Alaska. By the late 1970s, enough sophisticated features had been developed to give the system broad appeal in the United States, and communities began adopting it at the rate of 70 per year.

Latest figures show that 70% of the U.S. population and 35% of the geographic United States is covered by either basic or enhanced 9-1-1 service—the kind of emergency response system that figures so prominently in the television series. With basic 9-1-1, the call comes into an emergency answering center, which either dispatches the appropriate emergency personnel directly or transfers or relays the call to the appropriate agency, which then does the dispatching. The operator must elicit information from the caller about the address of the call.

With enhanced 9-1-1, the phone number, address, and name of the principal resident at the location automatically appear on a computer screen in front of the dispatcher when the call comes in.

Although it is impossible to estimate the numbers of lives and the amount of property saved because of the use of the 9-1-1 system, its obvious advantages lie in the reduced response time, better coordination among emergency agencies, and a higher degree of public confidence in the ability of its safety and emergency resources to serve its needs. "Rescue 911" strives to accurately portray how the system works, and what the "do's and don'ts" of emergency medical care are for citizen rescuers who are at the scene. The aim of this book is to give detailed advice about dealing with the accidents and medical emergencies you are most likely to encounter in and around your home. In many cases, this advice is illustrated with stories from the "Rescue 911" series that we believe capture the courage and the heroism with which so many people, just like you, automatically respond to these potentially disastrous events. We hope this book will give you the confidence and the information you need to deal with these situations with wisdom as well as compassion.

Thank you so much for making "Rescue 911" such an enormous success and for allowing us to continue to explore the highest dimensions of the human spirit in this very special way.

THE
RESCUE
911 ™
FAMILY
FIRST AID &
EMERGENCY
CARE BOOK

Asthma

Asthma is a condition caused by a gradual or sudden narrowing of the airway passages in the lungs, making breathing difficult, especially upon exhalation. This narrowing is the result of a spasm in the muscles that line these passages or the swelling of the passages (bronchi) themselves. Asthma is most common in children and young adults, and is often triggered by an allergic reaction to food, pollen, a drug, or some other substance to which the victim is highly sensitive. Infections of the bronchi (bronchitis), physical activity, cold weather, inhaled irritants, or emotional distress may also lead to an attack. Usually, someone with a history of asthma easily controls attacks with medication that stops the muscle spasm, opening the airway and allowing him or her to breathe more easily.

Sometimes, however, this is not possible, and the attack becomes a life-threatening emergency, as 16-year-old Angie Kenna of Milford, Ohio, discovered one harrowing night in November 1993.

1

Angie usually shared a room with her younger sister, Pam, but on November 12, Pam was staying at their father's house. Their mother, Beverly, went to bed early, while Angie stayed up to finish her homework. "Angie was diagnosed as an asthmatic at about the age of 5 or 6," Beverly said. "It's progressively gotten worse. When she gets short of breath, she can't walk any distance because she can't catch her breath enough to do so. She had had a period of 2 to 3 years where she hadn't had any serious attacks. With a severe asthma attack, the actual airway tree is so spasmed down that they're unable to breathe air in. They're going to die if they don't get help right away."

At 5:30 the next morning, Angie woke suddenly, gasping for air, in the grip of a severe asthma attack. She reached for her nebulizer to help her breathe, but the attack had progressed so far so quickly that it didn't work. Her bedroom door was closed, and she could not get enough air into her lungs to yell for help. She grabbed the phone near her bed and dialed 9-1-1.

Claremont County dispatcher Marcey Phillips took the call. "9-1-1 Emergency," she said.

"Help me," Angie gasped into the phone.

"What's the matter?" Phillips asked.

"Asthma," Angie managed to say.

"Okay, you're in apartment 27?" asked Phillips, who was able to trace the address of the call through the 9-1-1 system.

"Yes," came Angie's strained reply, followed by the sound of the phone falling to the floor.

"She just said 'asthma.' She couldn't talk enough to give me any information, but I knew where she lived through the 9-1-1 system. It appeared on my screen,"

Phillips said. "Okay, we have a person on the phone having a severe asthma attack," she reported to the police and to EMS (emergency medical services) personnel.

"Angie, are you still there?" Phillips asked, returning to the teenager's call. All she could hear in response was wheezing and coughing. "We're going to send a squad out, okay?" she went on. "Is there anybody with you?" There was no response.

"It scares you," she said, "because you don't know what's happening to her. The breathing machine got louder in the background. I could not hear her breathing at all. I lost contact with her, and there was nothing I could do to help her."

Miami Township police officer Gary Rausch had been on patrol less than 4 minutes away. "The dispatcher told me to proceed to an address with the report of a person having difficulty breathing," Rausch said. He knocked at the door of the Kennas' apartment, and Beverly answered it.

"To my surprise, there was a police officer at the door," she said. "I had no idea why he was there."

"Is everything okay here? Is there any problem here?" asked Rausch, as Beverly's boyfriend joined her at the door.

"You must have gotten a wrong number," Beverly said. "There's nothing wrong here."

"She said that there was no problem there. When I saw a boyfriend appear behind her, my initial suspicions were that it was a possible domestic quarrel of some sort," said Rausch. "If the people say there's no problem, I turn around and leave." Nonetheless, this time he went just a little further. "The dispatcher said she was actually talking to somebody and that the person was having trouble breathing and they lost contact," he said.

That was all that Beverly needed to hear. "Angie!" she cried, and raced to her daughter's room. "Right then I knew, if someone was having trouble breathing, who it was."

"It's my daughter! It's my daughter!" she yelled, after she reached Angie's side. "I was scared to death," she said. "Angie was unconscious and you could hear the mucus in her airways."

"She was turning blue," said Rausch, "so I advised dispatch to have them step it up."

Miami County paramedics Terry Robbins and Steve Monterosso arrived soon afterward. "The police officer said, 'Hurry up. It's a 16-year-old. She's not breathing,'" said Robbins. "Your heart kind of clamps up. I don't think you take a breath until you're inside there. With asthma, the air passages literally seal up. We were gong to have to open up her lungs or we were going to lose her."

"Just as I was putting an oral airway into her throat to put that tube into her, she clenched down her jaws, which made intubation almost impossible," said Monterosso. "I didn't want to lose what little airway we did have, and I just bagged her with a breathing bag.

"We're going to have to do something, Steve. We're not moving any air at all," said Robbins, who was watching Angie's chest for signs of motion. "She was so tight and closed up that as hard as we could squeeze that bag, we couldn't even force any air into her. We gave her some epinephrine, a little bit of air was now going in, but not enough to bring her around. You could literally watch her heart rate begin to slow down from lack of oxygen."

"I didn't believe that she would pull out of it," said Beverly.

University of Cincinnati Hospital flight doctor Sabrina Leach arrived and took charge of the scene. "I was very concerned because she was doing what we call posturing, which you see when somebody is not getting enough oxygen to her brain," Leach said. "If that continued, she could get permanent brain damage from that. She needed to have an airway. We went ahead and intubated her by inserting a breathing tube down her nose. We also went ahead and started giving her medication that is aerosolized and goes directly into the lungs. This was the most severe asthma case that I'd seen."

"We're going to be going to University Hospital," she told Beverly.

"It was so scary seeing her like that," Beverly said. "All I could think of was, would she survive this? She just looked so close to death."

Angie was flown to the hospital in an Air Care helicopter, and admitted to the emergency department under the care of Dr. Rashmi Kothari. "She was completely unresponsive and basically comatose," Kothari said. "She was young, which was in her favor, but it bothered me that she wasn't moving at all."

Angie's younger sister, Pam, and their father, David Kenna, joined Beverly at the hospital as soon as they heard what had happened. "I said, 'I love you, Angie,' and touched her hand so I could see if there was any reaction," David said. "And there was none."

"I was feeling very sad," said Pam. "I didn't know if something was wrong with her brain. But I knew she wouldn't die because she's a fighter."

Four days later, Angie was released from the hospital. Amazingly, she suffered no brain damage.

"It's made me want to stay closer to her," said Beverly. "Her asthma's still unstable at this point. She has new medication. She has a device that she carries with her so that if she has a problem, she can give herself a shot of adrenaline. I love her with all my heart. I'd do anything that I could to help her. If I could, I'd go through the asthma myself, but it's something that she has to do on her own, and all we can do is be there to encourage her."

"I used to be really embarrassed about my asthma," Angie said, "but then I realized that there would be times that I would have trouble in front of other people, and I couldn't hide it."

"It may never go away. It may always be there," said Beverly, "but she can get it under control. She can have a normal life."

"I love my sister and everything about her," Pam said. "She makes faces and jokes around a lot. If she wouldn't have made it, I'd miss her—all of her— being there. She's there for me whenever I need her."

"I want to thank everybody for what they did for her and how they helped her," Beverly said. "None of that would have happened, either, if she hadn't dialed 9-1-1."

"I've been told that she had only minutes—that it was that close," said David Kenna. "If the dispatcher had not seen the address on the screen, I'm almost positive that she would not have made it. I don't know if she knows it or not, but having almost lost her, there's almost nothing I wouldn't do at this point to protect her."

"Having asthma is hard," Angie said. "But it will never, never get the best of me."

Signs and Symptoms of Asthma (Any or All May Be Present):

➤ Difficulty in breathing. On exhalation, a wheezing or whistling sound is heard as air is forced out through narrow airways.
➤ A chest that appears larger than normal (particularly noticeable in small children) from the air trapped in the lungs
➤ Anxiety, tenseness, nervousness
➤ Coughing
➤ Sense of choking
➤ Possible vomiting
➤ Possible slight fever, if a concomitant illness is present
➤ Possible perspiration on the forehead
➤ If the victim is lying down when the attack occurs, he or she tries to sit upright and forward because this makes it easier to breathe.

Treatment for Asthma:

1. If this is the first time the victim is having an attack of suspected but as yet undiagnosed asthma, seek medical attention and report all details of the attack. Calm and reassure the victim; emotional distress may aggravate the situation. A child may be particularly frightened by the experience and in need of comfort.
2. If the victim is known to have asthma and attacks have occurred before, give him or her the pre-

scribed medications, following the instructions on the container. Report the attack to the victim's physician.

3. Do not try to get the victim to lie down.
4. Call EMS personnel *immediately* if the signs and symptoms continue and any of the following occurs:

   - The victim does not improve with medication.
   - There is difficulty in breathing or an inability to exhale; breathing becomes barely audible.
   - The victim cannot cough.
   - There is an increased bluish tinge to the skin.
   - The pulse rate increases to more than 120 beats per minute.
   - There is increased anxiety.
   - *The victim tries to pull up the shoulders and chin to expand the chest.* This signals that the victim may be close to respiratory failure and could collapse.

Bites and Stings

The common sources of injected poisons are stings and bites from insects and other animals (see also poisoning, p. 257. In addition to those venoms that are generally poisonous, there are some to which certain people have extreme allergic reactions, which can be fatal. This life-threatening condition is called anaphylaxis. In addition, there are insects that carry diseases and those that transmit toxins picked up from poisonous substances on which they have been feeding or with which they have come into contact. The most common stinging insects are bumblebees, honeybees, wasps, hornets, yellow jackets, and fire ants.

Treatment of Insect Stings:

1. Examine the area to see if the stinger is left in the skin. (This is usually the case with honeybee stings.)
2. If it is, remove it to prevent further poisoning. Do this by gently scraping the skin with a knife blade, plastic card edge, or fingernail. The venom

sac will often still be attached to the stinger. *Do not* try to remove the stinger with tweezers, since any squeezing may compress the venom sac and send more poison into the body.

3. Wash the area with soap and water.
4. Place ice wrapped in a cloth or cold compresses on the sting area to decrease the absorption and spread of venom and to reduce the pain and swelling.
5. Check the victim periodically for an allergic reaction.

Anaphylaxis, or *anaphylactic shock,* an extreme allergic, whole-body reaction to a substance, is rare but life threatening, and can occur in response to insect bites or stings, especially if the victim has been bitten or stung previously. Other common causes are certain foods or food additives, particularly shellfish, berries, and sulfites; medications such as penicillin; and inhaled substances such as dust and pollen. Sensitivity reactions happen suddenly, within seconds or minutes after contact with the substance. Death from anaphylaxis, which can happen within minutes, usually occurs because the victim's breathing is severely impaired. A person who has this extreme degree of sensitivity to such substances should wear a medical alert tag. Some people who are aware of their vulnerability to this kind of allergic reaction carry medication with them to reverse it.

Signs and Symptoms of Anaphylactic Shock

➤ Swelling and redness at the site of the bite or sting

- ➤ Severe swelling in other parts of the body, such as the eyes, lip, and tongue
- ➤ Hives or a hivelike rash
- ➤ Severe itching
- ➤ Coughing and wheezing
- ➤ Difficulty in breathing, which can progress to an obstructed airway as the throat and tongue swell
- ➤ Tightness in the chest area
- ➤ Stomach cramps
- ➤ Nausea and vomiting
- ➤ Weakness
- ➤ Anxiety
- ➤ Dizziness
- ➤ Lightheadedness
- ➤ Possible bluish tinge to the skin
- ➤ Collapse
- ➤ Possible unconsciousness

Although anaphylaxis is rare, it is especially dangerous because it can strike suddenly, and the victim is often unaware of his own allergic condition. This is what happened on a serene summer's day in 1993 to 36-year-old Eugean Heiney of Essex, Connecticut.

On the afternoon of August 7, Eugean (or Gean, as his friends call him), an off-duty police officer, was trying to do some clean-up work on a house he had just finished building in a neighboring town. Gean stopped by his parents' house first to pick up his younger brother Erik so he could help. Erik, who was 27 at the time, is a Down's syndrome victim, and a Special Olympics athlete.

"Gean was going to be moving some boxes from

his apartment up to his new home," their mother explained. "Erik doesn't get to spend as much time as he would like with Gean, so he was eager to go. One thing about Erik and other Down's syndrome children is that they only see the good side of people. They never see anything bad about anyone."

"He's more or less taken it up on his own to be competitive," said Erik's father, "whether it's the Special Olympics or in his volunteer work with the fire department or on the job. He's a special guy. That's it. He's just special."

"There was a pile of wood scraps that the builders had tossed out by the side of the driveway," said Mrs. Heiney, "and Gean decided that they should move that lumber out of the way, down the hill."

Erik positioned himself on the top of the hill, by the wood, and began tossing it down to Gean, stationed below. "I love that—tossing it down," Erik said.

All of a sudden, Gean began slapping at his legs. He had unwittingly disturbed a nest of yellow jackets, who had repaid his mistake by stinging him more that 20 times on the legs. He dashed up the hill to escape his swarming tormentors. "There's bees down there," he said, still panting for breath, warning Erik not to go down the hill.

"Are you all right?" Erik asked.

"Yes, I'm all right, but don't go down there. I'm going to sit down in the garage for a moment," Gean replied.

"Are you okay?" Erik asked when his brother came back from the garage.

"I'm just hot," Gean answered, and then he began coughing and wheezing.

"Are you okay?" Erik asked again, his concern mounting.

"I'm okay," Gean assured him, but Erik noticed that he was red and sweating profusely. He asked his brother if he didn't think he should go to the clinic, but Gean said no, asserting again that he would be all right. Then he said that he would lie down in the truck for a minute.

Erik looked in on him a little while later, and asked his brother again if he were okay and if he wanted to go to the hospital. "No, I don't want to go to the hospital," Gean said emphatically. He got out of the truck and collapsed face down a few feet away.

"Are you okay?" Erik asked once more, hoping that his brother would agree to get some help.

"Yes, I'm okay," Gean stubbornly insisted. "Just help me get back into the truck." When he was back in the truck, Erik checked his forehead and found that it was very warm. Again, he urged his brother to go to the clinic. "I just have to lie down," Gean insisted.

"You'll be okay?" Erik asked anxiously.

"Why don't you go on. I'll be all right," Gean said. Once Erik had left his side, however, Gean tried to use the radio in his car to call police headquarters, but got no response. Panicked by his deteriorating condition, he called out to Erik. When his brother rushed up to the truck, he told him to go to the nearest house and call for help. Erik dashed off down the hill, realizing how serious the situation had become from the tone of his brother's voice and the symptoms he had observed. He reached the house of Hayne Bayless.

"I opened the door and there was this guy there,"

said Bayless, "and he was trying to tell me something was wrong."

"Up on the hill—stung by bees," Erik said.

"Even though it was really hard to understand his individual words," Bayless said, "It was not hard to understand that something was really wrong."

Bayless called 9-1-1, and local fire-department and ambulance volunteers were immediately dispatched to the scene, along with Middlesex Hospital paramedic Phil Coco, who happened to be a good friend of Gean's. "As I pulled up, Erik came down to the truck and told me that someone had been stung by a bee," Coco said. "He didn't indicate exactly who it was at the time. A volunteer of the Essex Fire Department had begun care. I performed a visual assessment and realized that the situation was life threatening, and *then* I realized that the patient was Gean Heiney. Anaphylactic shock begins very rapidly and generally speaking, there are only a very few minutes from the time of onset until death. To reverse the situation, we needed to establish some large-bore IVs [intravenous tubes] and get some fluid going, to restore blood pressure, and we also—more acutely—needed to administer epinephrine and Benedryl."

"I said, 'God, let my brother live. Don't let my brother die. I love him,' and then I started crying," said Erik. In spite of the emotional impact of the scene, Erik was able to coordinate efforts to get his brother into the ambulance. "Get better," Erik said to Gean as Gean was being loaded into the stretcher for transport to the hospital.

"I'll take you down to the clinic and you can watch him there," said Coco to Erik soothingly.

Gean was treated for his allergic reaction to the

stings and was released the same day, although cases of this severity are often kept under observation for 24 hours. "I remember Erik standing behind me, and saying, 'Is everybody ready? One, two, three,' as they lifted me up to put me in the ambulance," Gean said. "I remember feeling this swell of pride that he was standing at my head, that he was giving the commands, and that he wasn't going to leave me. And as I was being carried to the ambulance I heard him say, 'Don't worry, I'm not going to leave you—I love you.'"

"When Erik was first born, I'll never forget it," said his father. "It was December 8, and the doctor called me up the next day and he said, 'I'm going to have to tell you your son is a mongoloid.' I couldn't even say the word. That was 27 years ago. Today, I'm proud to be able to say that I have a Down's syndrome son."

"I think that regardless of anyone's age or handicap that they should be trained what to do in an emergency," Coco says, "because when an emergency strikes, you would be surprised what little kids and handicapped people are able to do when they know somebody's life is on the line. And I think Erik is a perfect example of that."

"I'm not surprised at all that Erik was able to handle the situation," said his mother. "It's just like him. I've heard people say that they wonder why God put such people on this earth. Well, this incident is just another example of how capable these handicapped people are."

"Gean is my friend and a police officer, and I know he knows what anaphylactic shock is," said Phil Coco, "but people go through denial—and in this case, denial almost cost him his life."

Gean now carries an epinephrine kit with him at all times. "Anaphylactic shock really isn't anything to fool with," he says. "There's nothing you can do to help yourself except to get to a medical facility right away. I remember having that conscious thought that Erik would be able to help me, and I had no doubt about that. I owe him—I owe him big time."

"I love my brother," Erik said. "I kept my fingers crossed. Nice big hug and a happy ending. I say, 'God, thank you. You answered my prayers.'"

Treatment for Allergic Reaction to Insect Stings:

Be aware that any allergic reaction can turn into anaphylaxis, and observe the victim carefully if an unusual inflammation or rash appears immediately after contact with the source of injection.

1. Assess breathing and keep an airway open (see p. 160).
2. Remove any stinger left in the skin as described above.
3. If the person has difficulty breathing or complains that his or her throat is closing, call EMS personnel immediately. Help the person into the most comfortable position for breathing.
4. If the person is carrying an anaphylaxis kit or if an emergency kit for insect stings is available, help him or her to find and take the medicine in the kit.
5. Seek medical attention promptly.

If you have a history of sensitivity to insect bites, avoid situations in which you may be stung. In the event you are stung, be prepared with a plan, which should include always carrying your medications, wearing Medic Alert identification and notifying those with you about your allergy.

Bites and Stings of Spiders, Centipedes, Tarantulas, and Scorpions

The bites and stings of spiders, centipedes, tarantulas, and scorpions can cause alarming symptoms, and their effects are usually much more severe than those of the stinging insects mentioned above. Spider bites generally consist of two pinpoint punctures of the skin that produce local swelling and redness with a smarting, burning pain.

It is important to learn about the potentially dangerous spiders in your area. Spiders are nonaggressive, and people are generally bitten because the spider has been provoked by rough handling or traumatized by a surprise invasion of its territory.

Both the *black widow spider* and the *brown recluse spider* live in most parts of the United States. They prefer dark, out-of-the-way places where there is small likelihood that they will be disturbed. Bites usually occur on the hands and arms of people reaching into places like woodpiles, rock piles, and brush piles or rummaging in dark garages, basements, and attics. Frequently, the victim will not know that he or she has been bitten until the symptoms develop. Though both types of bites can be fatal, the bite of the black widow spider is the more painful and often the more deadly of the two. Its venom, in fact, is more toxic than that of a rattlesnake.

The *black widow spider* is moderately large and glossy black with very fine hairs over the body that give it a silky appearance. There is a characteristic bright red or crimson marking in the shape of an hourglass on the underside of its body. Only the female is poisonous. Black widow spider bites are particularly harmful to small children, the elderly, and the chronically ill.

Signs and Symptoms of a Black Widow Spider Bite (Any or All May Be Present):

➤ Slight redness and swelling around the bite
➤ Sharp pain around the bite
➤ Profuse sweating
➤ Nausea and possible vomiting
➤ Stomach cramps or hard, rigid abdomen
➤ Possible muscle cramps in other parts of the body
➤ Tightness in the chest and difficulty in breathing and talking
➤ Neurological symptoms or weakness

The *brown recluse ("fiddle back") spider* is light brown with a darker brown violin-shaped marking on the top of its body. It injects a venom that causes a limited destruction of red blood cells and certain other harmful alterations in the blood. Its bite causes severe, deep, irreversible damage to the tissue around the bite area and is particularly harmful to very young children.

Signs and Symptoms of a Brown Recluse Spider Bite (Any or All May Be Present):

➤ The victim feels a stinging sensation at the time of the bite.
➤ Redness occurs, disappearing later as a blister forms.

➤ If the bite is not treated promptly, pain becomes more severe during the following 8 hours.
➤ Over the next 48 hours, chills, fever, nausea, vomiting, joint pains, and possibly a rash appear.
➤ Destruction of tissue forms an open ulcer.

Treatment for Black Widow and Brown Recluse Spider Bites:

1. Maintain an open airway and restore breathing if necessary (see p. 160).
2. Keep the bitten area lower than the victim's heart.
3. Place ice wrapped in cloth or cold compresses on the bitten area.
4. Seek medical attention promptly, preferably at the nearest hospital emergency department. If possible, take the spider with you. Professionals will clean the wound and give medication to reduce the pain and inflammation. There is an antivenin available for black widow bites.

Tarantulas are large spiders with very hairy bodies and legs, usually found in the Southwest. Those native to the United States are not poisonous, although a severe allergic reaction is possible, but those that travel into the country with imported fruit may be. There may be no pain experienced at the time of the bite, but extreme local pain, redness, and swelling can develop later.

Treatment for Tarantula Bites:

1. Wash the area with soap and water.

2. Place ice wrapped in cloth or cold compresses on the bite area.
3. Soothing lotions such as calamine may be useful in reducing discomfort.
4. If a severe reaction occurs, seek medical attention promptly.

Scorpions also live in the dry regions of the U.S. Southwest, and most U.S. species do not inject a venom that is harmful to humans. A scorpion looks like a small lobster, with a set of pincers and a stinger located in its tail, which arches over its back. They are found under rocks, logs, and the bark of certain trees and are most active at night. The scorpion's sting may result in local swelling and discoloration, similar to a wasp sting, and may sometimes cause allergic reactions. The sting of the more dangerous species, which is extremely harmful to very young children, contains a poison that acts on the nervous system. It causes little or no swelling or discoloration but may result in the following signs and symptoms.

Signs and Symptoms of Poisonous Scorpion Stings (Any or All May Be Present):

➤ Severe burning pain or tingling at the site of the sting
➤ Nausea and vomiting
➤ Numbness and tingling in the affected area
➤ Possible spasm of jaw muscles, making opening of the mouth difficult
➤ Stomach pain
➤ Twitching and spasm of affected muscles

➤ Shock
➤ Convulsions
➤ Possible coma

Treatment for Poisonous Scorpion Stings:

1. Call EMS personnel, who can transport the victim to a medical facility where an antivenin is available. While waiting for EMS personnel to arrive:
2. Maintain an open airway. Restore breathing and circulation if necessary (see pp. 160 and 229).
3. Keep the bitten area lower than the victim's heart.
4. Place ice wrapped in cloth or cold compresses on the bitten area.
5. Keep the victim calm and quiet.
6. Treat for shock (see p. 305) if necessary.

Snake Bites

There are four kinds of poisonous snakes in the United States, three of which are of the type known as the pit viper. These are rattlesnakes, copperheads, and water moccasins (also known as cottonmouths). The fourth is the coral snake. Rattlesnakes can be found all over the country, while copperheads and water moccasins live mostly in the southeast and south central parts of the country and coral snakes primarily inhabit the southeast. While about 8,000 people are bitten annually in the United States, fewer than 12 die each year from snake bites. Rattlesnakes account for most snake bites and nearly all fatalities from snake bites. Death gener-

----

ally occurs because the victim has an allergic reaction to the venom or a weakened overall condition or because much time passes before the victim receives medical care.

It is important to learn what snakes live in your region or the area you're visiting. Be aware that even a dead snake can release venom. When walking outdoors, wear long pants and boots, since the most common targets are the ankles and feet. Walk only on clear paths and carry a walking stick.

The rattlesnake, copperhead, and water moccasin have the characteristic triangular-shaped head and deep pits (which are poison sacs) located between the nostrils and the eyes of pit vipers. They have slitlike eyes rather than the rounded eyes of nonpoisonous snakes (the exception to this being the coral snake, which also has rounded eyes). They have long fangs that leave distinctive marks followed by a row of teeth marks. The rattlesnake is also characterized by the rattles at the end of its tail, and the water moccasin by a white coloring inside its mouth.

Signs and Symptoms of Pit Viper Bites (Any and All May Be Present):

➤ Severe pain
➤ Rapid swelling
➤ Discoloration of the skin around the bite
➤ Weakness
➤ Nausea and vomiting
➤ Difficulty in breathing
➤ Blurring vision

➤ Convulsions
➤ Shock

Treatment for Pit Viper Bites:

1. Call EMS professionals.
2. Keep the victim lying down and quiet, with the wounded part lower than the rest of the body if possible.
3. Remove all rings, watches, and bracelets from the extremity in case of swelling.
4. Wash the wound if possible.
5. Immobilize a wounded limb or digit with a splint.
6. Treat for shock if necessary (see p. 305).
7. If the victim must be transported, carry him or her or have him or her walk slowly.
8. Monitor vital signs during transportation.
9. If it is clear that the victim cannot get professional medical care within 30 minutes and a snake-bite kit is available, consider using it to suction the wound.
10. *Do not* give the victim anything by mouth.
11. *Do not,* regardless of what you may have otherwise heard or read:

   • Apply ice—this can cause as much harm as good
   • Cut the wound—this can further harm the victim and has not been demonstrated to remove any significant amount of venom
   • Suck the venom from the wound using your mouth

- Apply a tourniquet—this could severely reduce blood flow to the limb, resulting in loss of the limb
- Use electric shock—this has not been shown to conclusively affect the poison and can be dangerous

The *coral snake,* a member of the cobra family, has the rounded eyes of nonpoisonous snakes and fangs through which its poison is delivered. It also has distinctive markings of red, yellow, and black rings the entire length of its body. The yellow rings are narrow and always separate the red and the black rings. An old rhyme for remembering this pattern is: "Red on yellow will kill a fellow/Red on black won't hurt Jack." The coral snake is smaller than the pit vipers and always has a black nose. Some signs and symptoms of snake bite may not occur immediately.

Signs and Symptoms of Coral Snake Bites (Any or All May Be Present):

➤ Slight pain and swelling at the location of the bite
➤ Blurred vision
➤ Drooping eyelids
➤ Difficulty speaking
➤ Heavy drooling
➤ Drowsiness
➤ Heavy sweating
➤ Nausea and vomiting
➤ Difficulty breathing
➤ Paralysis
➤ Shock

Treatment for Coral Snake Bites:

1. Call EMS personnel or transport the victim to the nearest hospital emergency department. If possible, call ahead to notify the hospital of the poisonous snake bite and the type of snake so that antivenin can be ready.
2. Quickly wash the affected area.
3. Immobilize the affected limb or digit with a splint.
4. Keep the victim quiet.
5. *Do not:*

   - Tie off the bite area
   - Apply ice or cold compresses
   - Give the victim food or alcoholic beverages

Treatment for a Nonpoisonous Snake Bite:

1. Keep the bitten area below the level of the victim's heart.
2. Clean the area thoroughly with soap and water.
3. Put a bandage or clean cloth over the wound.
4. Seek medical attention, as medication to prevent infection or a tetanus shot may be necessary.

Bites by Mammals (Warm-Blooded Animals)

The bite of any wild or domestic animal can result in serious infection as well as tissue damage. Cat scratches can also be dangerous, causing cat-scratch fever, a glandular infection. Tetanus is a common risk, but the most serious possible outcome is rabies, which is transmitted through the saliva of diseased animals such as skunks, raccoons, bats, cats, dogs, cattle, squirrels, and foxes. If not treated, rabies is fatal.

Rabid animals (animals infected with rabies) may act in abnormal ways. For example, nocturnal animals, such as raccoons and opossums, may become active in the daytime. A wild animal, which usually avoids humans, may not run away when you approach. Rabid animals may salivate, appear partially paralyzed, or act irritable, aggressive, or strangely quiet. Do not pet or feed wild animals and do not touch the body of a dead wild animal. Keep your pets' rabies immunizations up to date.

In the past, treatment for rabies consisted of a long series of painful vaccine injections, with multiple unpleasant side effects, to build up immunity to the disease. Treatment today requires fewer injections with more mild side effects.

With the exception of rabid animals, most animals will attack only if provoked. To avoid problems, however, it is best not to leave a child alone with an animal, including your household pet. Warn your children to be cautious around pets they don't know.

Treatment for Animal Bites:

1. Try to get the victim away from the animal without endangering yourself. *Do not* try to capture or restrain the animal, but try to observe it clearly so it can be described to the emergency dispatcher, who will notify the animal-control authorities.
2. Control bleeding (see p. 37). If the bleeding is

severe, do not clean the wound. This will be properly done at a medical facility.

3. If the bleeding is not severe, wash the wound with sterile water or saline solution, if available, or soap and running water for at least 5 minutes to wash out any dangerous microorganisms.

4. Dress and bandage the wound.

5. Take the victim to a medical facility as quickly as possible.

6. Notify local authorities about the animal; if possible, give description and location.

Bleeding

If the tissues of the body do not receive blood, they will die from lack of oxygen. The loss of 2 pints of blood—8% to 10% of the body's total—by an adult is considered serious. The loss of 3 pints can be very dangerous if it occurs over a relatively short period of time—1 to 2 hours. The loss of 4 pints or more will necessitate blood transfusions to prevent death.

There are certain points in the body where fatal bleeding can occur in a very short period of time. If either of the two principle blood vessels in the neck, the arms, or the thighs is cut, the loss of blood may prove fatal in 3 minutes or less. If one of the main trunk blood vessels in the chest and abdomen is ruptured, death can occur in less than 30 seconds.

When the body loses a large quantity of blood, it goes into a state of physical shock, in which blood is shunted to vital organs, most bodily functions slow down, and all bodily processes are affected.

EXTERNAL BLEEDING

Minor external bleeding—by far the most common sort in household injuries—will usually stop by itself when the blood clots, within 10 minutes.

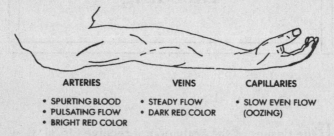

ARTERIES	VEINS	CAPILLARIES
• SPURTING BLOOD	• STEADY FLOW	• SLOW EVEN FLOW
• PULSATING FLOW	• DARK RED COLOR	(OOZING)
• BRIGHT RED COLOR		

Bleeding Characteristics

If the bleeding is caused by damage to a large blood vessel, or one in which the blood is under a lot of pressure, clotting may not occur and the bleeding may become severe and even life threatening.

There are three identifiable kinds of external bleeding: bleeding from an artery, bleeding from a vein, and bleeding from capillaries. An artery has been cut when bright red blood spurts from a wound. A vein has been cut when dark red blood flows from a wound in a steady stream. When blood oozes slowly from a wound, capillaries have been cut, and there is usually little cause for alarm about blood loss. When a large area of skin surface is involved, there may be some threat of infection.

On March 13, 1992, Joetta Sharrard of Grants Pass, Oregon, learned how vulnerable children can be to injuries that cause severe, life-threatening bleeding. That afternoon, she uncharacteristically left her three sons and one of the boys' visiting friends alone in the house, watching cartoons on television, as she went to run an errand. "I normally don't leave my kids at home alone," she said, "but I had to do this errand, and none of the kids wanted to come with me. I thought to myself, 'They'll be okay here, and I'm only going to be gone a few minutes.'"

"I don't want any rough stuff while I'm gone," she cautioned them, leaving her 11-year-old son, Michael, in charge.

Soon after she left, Michael, Evan, and 7-year-old Ben, Michael's brother, decided to go outside and play tag. "I told my friend, Evan, that I wanted to do something else because the cartoons were getting boring," Michael said.

In the yard next door, 45-year-old John Miller heard the excited sounds of the boys playing as he watched his father, Clarence, repair a wound in an old tree. "My father had asked me to come over and help him do some odd jobs on some of his rental houses," John said. "I listened to the horseplay, and it wasn't anything that alarmed me. I'm used to boys carrying on like that."

"We were playing tag and I was it," Michael said. "I went after Ben, and it just happened, real quick." Ben had run up the steps leading to their back door. When Michael reached out to tag him from behind, Ben lost his balance and his arms went crashing through the nonsafety glass of one of the door panes. Reflexively pulling them back through the jagged glass, he slashed both his arms badly.

The Millers heard the sound of breaking glass, and then terrifying screams.

"I'm dying, Michael," Ben screamed, as blood streamed down his arms.

"All I saw was blood everywhere," Michael said, "and then I started screaming 'Oh my God! Oh my God.'"

The Millers ran next door to help, and John instructed Michael to call 9-1-1. "I rushed to Ben," John Miller said. "I had never seen such an ugly cut in my life. I had received a lot of training in first aid in the navy. And so we elevated his arms and applied the pressure. I knew that if we did not stop the bleeding, this boy was going to die on us, and I was not going to let that happen." John and his father each took one of Michael's arms and, raising it above the level of his heart, applied direct pressure to the wounds and pressed on the axillary pressure point above the elbow, pushing the artery against the bone to cut off the flow of blood to the rest of the arm.

"In the back of my mind I was afraid that this lad was not going to live," John said. "In a way, I was angry about that thought. I've always thought it unfair of fate to arrange it so that a child has to die. I decided that fate was going to have a fight."

Sue Illions, the dispatcher who handled the response to Michael's 9-1-1 call, heard the heartrending sound of a child, helpless with fear. "The first thing I heard when the call came in was a child screaming 'Oh my God!' she said. "That sets our blood going. You want to reach out and grab this child and say 'It's going to be okay. I'm going to help you through this.'"

As John and Clarence tended to Ben's wounds, Sue tried to get more specific information about the situation from Michael. Then she told him to wrap his brother's wounds with a towel or other clean cloth and apply direct pressure to the cuts by pressing the cloths down on them, but not squeezing too hard. Michael left the phone for a minute to relay the message to John, who got the towels and did the bandaging.

Back on the phone, Michael continued to sob hysterically, while Sue tried to comfort and reassure him. "Michael, Michael," she said, "you're doing okay. Your brother's not going to die. He just cut his arms and we have an ambulance on the way. I know blood is a very scary thing," she told Michael, "but if you get upset, your brother will get upset."

"Imagine being 11 and seeing all this blood covering your brother's arms," she later said.

"I was really scared," Michael said. "I was in so much shock, I couldn't move. I just didn't want him to die."

Just then Joetta returned, and heard in a panic Michael's account of what had happened. Sue told Michael repeatedly and insistently to put his now-distraught mother, who had run out to be with Ben, on the phone.

"There were two men standing out there and they wouldn't let me see him," said Joetta, referring to Clarence and John. "That was real hard for me. I just wanted to hold him and they wouldn't let me see him."

Michael finally persuaded his mother to come back in the house and get on the phone with the dispatcher, who tried to calm her down and give her a realistic assessment of the situation. "Hi!" Sue said, counteracting Joetta's hysteria with a firm, matter-of-fact manner. "You're all right. Let's not get all excited here, or you're going to scare Benjamin. Listen to me! Listen to me! Listen to me!" Sue said emphatically, over

Joetta's sobs. "You're doing just fine. Michael called 9-1-1, and we've got an ambulance that should be there any second."

"I can't breathe," gasped Joetta.

"You need to slow down. Do you hear the ambulance yet?" Sue asked.

"I hear it, but I don't think they can find my house," said Joetta, still in the grip of panic.

"You need to calm down, because this is not going to help anyone. The ambulance is right on the corner. Now they're right there," said Sue.

"Will they let me go with him?" Joetta asked, desperately.

"Sure they will," Sue told her. "They're on the scene now. I'm going to keep you on the line until I'm sure that you're calmed down a little. It's not going to help the paramedics if you guys are all upset there. Everything's going to be all right. What's your name?"

"Joetta."

"Okay, Joetta, you need to calm down for everybody. How's Benjamin doing?"

"He's calm," Joetta replied. "He looked really pale, though."

"Okay," Sue said.

"But there's so much blood on the table!"

"Okay. A little blood goes a long way," Sue said knowledgeably. "We've got the ambulance there, and they're going to check on him. I don't want you to get upset, because that will upset Benjamin. You're the mom, and Mom has got to be strong right now."

"I'm a wimp!" Joetta said, miserably.

"You're not a wimp!" Sue said, both emphatically and sympathetically. "Will you be strong for me now?"

"Yes," Joetta answered, more calmly.

"Will you take care of yourself?" Sue asked, unwilling to end the conversation until she felt certain that Joetta had regained control of herself.

"I'm able to," Joetta said, still a little unsurely.

"You're not a wimp," Sue repeated. "You be strong. Okay?"

"Okay," Joetta answered, more assuredly.

"All right. Go for it!" Sue said, and hung up.

"When you hang up after a high emotional call such as that one," Sue said, "the frustration is so high that you want to just unplug and go over there and make sure that everything's okay. We just have to hang up the phone and wonder."

The paramedics on the scene assessed Ben's condition. They discovered that the wound on his left arm was particularly bad, and that Ben had no sensation in the fingers of his left hand and was unable to move some of them. "Usually, children don't handle injuries of this nature well," said paramedic Marvin Aaron. "Because Benjamin kept a cool head and because he was such a nice boy, my heart just went out to him."

"He didn't have any color to his face at all, and his lips were white," Joetta said. "And he just kept saying to me, 'Mom, I can't feel my arms. I can't feel my arms.' While he was telling me that I was wondering, 'God, will he ever be able to use them again?'"

Benjamin was taken to the hospital, where he was examined by plastic surgeon Ronald Worland. "When Ben came in the hand was alive, so I knew that one of the arteries at least was functional," Dr. Worland said. "The surgery involved repairing nine tendons to the hand, both of the major nerves and, of course, the skin defect, which had occurred when he fell through the glass. The work of the surgery is done through a microscope. Because the stitches are so small, we never know if the nerves or the tendons will work. We had a probable 70% chance of the nerves functioning."

"I didn't think he'd ever be able to use his arm again," Joetta said. "You know—do those things again, be a little boy, jump and run and swing on monkey bars. I never realized until that point how you take for granted being able to do things like that. An arm is a precious thing."

After a year of grueling physical therapy, Ben completely regained the use of his arms.

"It was really scary," Ben said. "I didn't think I'd be able to use my arms again. But I feel fine. I can use my hand. I can swing on the monkey bars."

"The first time he ran and grabbed a monkey bar, and swung on it, all of us cried," Joetta said. "It was a magic moment. When I see him out playing, my heart just leaps—and the phrase 'Hold me, Mom' takes on a whole new meaning. Just give me a hug—with both arms. That's all I want."

"When he got home, every night I slept by him on the floor because I wanted to be with him the whole time," Michael said. "I love my brother a lot. I'm just glad he's alive. If he was dead, I don't know what I would do. I don't know if I could live if he died. I would hope that nothing else bad will happen, and everything will go good in our lives."

"He could have died—he could have bled to death," said Charles Sharrard, Ben's grateful father, "if it weren't for Michael and the Millers and 9-1-1 and the paramedics and the doctors. I just thank them very much, because they helped save Benjamin's life. He's a walking miracle."

Control of external bleeding is usually very simple, and generally done by applying direct pressure to the open wound with the hand. This permits normal clotting to occur. In cases of severe bleeding, the appearance of the wound and the emotional state of the victim may seem alarming. It is important to remember that a small amount of blood can seem like a great deal.

___

Control of External Bleeding:

1. *Direct Pressure.* Place a thick layer of sterile gauze or the cleanest material available (a towel, a washcloth, a dishcloth, a T-shirt, strips of sheeting, or a handkerchief may be used) against the bleeding part and apply firm pressure with the palm of your hand until a cover bandage can be applied. If no cloth is available, have the victim apply pressure with his or her hand. If this is not possible, use your own hand directly on the wound.
2. *Elevation.* If a limb is bleeding, try to elevate it above the level of the heart to reduce the pressure of the flow.
3. *Pressure bandage.* Keep hand pressure on the wound until the bleeding slows. If blood soaks through the original cloth or pad, do *not* remove it. Place another cloth or pad on top of it. Apply a pressure bandage to hold the pad or cloth in place. Put the midpoint of the bandage directly over the compress. Holding it in place there with one hand—or having the victim hold it in place—pull steadily on both ends as you wrap them around. Then tie the ends together in a knot di-

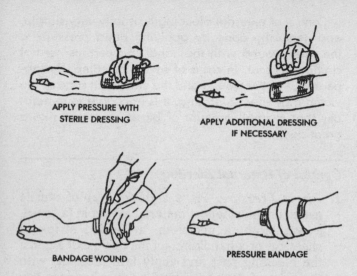

**APPLY PRESSURE WITH
STERILE DRESSING**

**APPLY ADDITIONAL DRESSING
IF NECESSARY**

BANDAGE WOUND

PRESSURE BANDAGE

Direct Pressure

rectly over the wound. Do not tie them so tightly that you cut off circulation. If bleeding continues, the bandage is not applying enough pressure. Use your hand over the bandage to apply more pressure, or apply a second bandage *over* the original dressing.

Nosebleeds

A nosebleed can be caused by a blow to the nose, scratching the nose, repeated blowing of the nose (which irritates the mucous membrane, especially in cold weather when indoor heated air dries out the nasal passages), or by an infection. In children, nosebleeds are not serious, but nosebleeds in the elderly may be dangerous and require treatment in a hospital emergency room.

Treatment for Nosebleeds:

1. Keep the victim seated and leaning forward with the mouth open, so that blood or clots will not close off the airway.
2. Gently pinch the affected nostril closed and keep it closed for approximately 15 minutes. Release slowly. Do not allow the victim to blow or touch the nose. If bleeding persists, pinch the nostrils closed for another 5 minutes.
3. It may be helpful to apply pressure beneath the nose, above the lip. If these measures do not succeed in controlling the bleeding, it may in rare cases be caused by a disease such as high blood pressure, in which case the victim should see a physician. If the nose is injured, the victim should be examined for possible facial fractures. If a skull fracture is suspected, and clear liquid (cerebrospinal fluid) is mixed with the blood, do *not* try to stop the bleeding, since this might increase pressure on the brain. Treat for a fractured skull (see p. 214).

Tips for Preventing External Bleeding:

- Make sure that all doors containing glass, including shower doors, use safety glass that will not shatter if broken.

- Keep sharp objects like scissors, knives, and razor blades out of the reach of children.

- Use plastic or paper drinking glasses in the bathroom and with small children.

- Do not allow children to take tableware made of glass out of the kitchen or dining room.

Open Wounds

A wound that bleeds externally, in which the skin has been broken, is called an *open wound*. When the skin is unbroken, it protects the body's tissues from external bacteria. Even a small break in the skin may allow them to enter, causing infection. Sometimes the flow of blood will wash out the bacteria carried into the body by the object creating the wound, but some types of wounds do not bleed freely enough to do this. All open wounds should receive prompt medical attention. Sometimes, as in the case of head injuries, they are the only external signs of a more serious injury, such as skull fracture.

There are six main types of open wounds: abrasions, lacerations, incisions, avulsions, amputations, and punctures.

1. *Abrasion.* This is a rubbing or scraping away of the skin, as when a child falls and scrapes his or her hands or knees. It is usually painful, though the bleeding is not serious. The wound should be thoroughly washed with soap and water to prevent infection.
2. *Incision.* This is a wound with smooth edges, caused by a sharp cutting edge like a knife, a razor, scissors, or broken glass. Incisions usually bleed freely and, depending on how deep they are and the structures involved, may bleed pro-

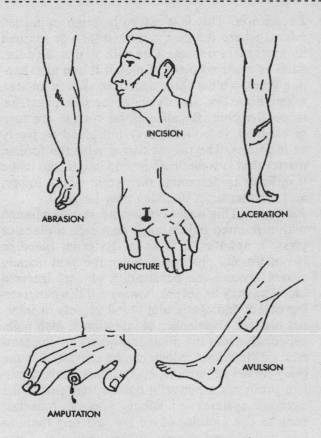

INCISION

ABRASION

LACERATION

PUNCTURE

AVULSION

AMPUTATION

Classification of Open Wounds

fusely. Deep incisions can also affect layers of fat and muscle and damage both blood vessels and nerves. If there is enough nerve damage, feeling in the area may be destroyed and the incision may not be painful.

3. *Laceration.* This is a cut with rough or jagged edges, where the flesh has been torn or mashed by machinery or something with an uneven edge, such as a jagged piece of metal. It can also happen when a blunt force splits the skin in an area where bone lies directly under the skin's surface, as on the chin. Because blood vessels are torn or mashed, lacerations may not bleed as freely as incisions. The ragged tissue, with the foreign matter that is sometimes ground into it, can make it difficult to determine the extent of the injury, and the danger of infection may be great.

4. *Puncture.* This occurs when the skin is pierced with a pointed object, such as a nail, a piece of glass, a splinter, or a knife. External bleeding is not usually profuse, because the skin usually closes around the penetrating object. Internal bleeding may be severe, however, if the penetrating object damages major blood vessels or internal organs. The danger of infection is also high, especially from the microorganism causing tetanus, or "lockjaw," which can be carried into the body by the penetrating object. This microorganism produces a powerful poison that enters the nervous system and affects specific muscles, such as the muscles of the jaw, causing them to contract beyond the control of the victim. Once the tetanus bacteria reach the nervous system, the results are irreversible. An object that remains embedded in a puncture wound is called an impaled object, and it must be treated with special caution (see Special Treatment for Specific Open Wounds, p. 52).

5. *Avulsion.* A portion of the skin and sometimes

other soft tissue is torn partially or wholly away, leaving a completely exposed area or one on which the tissue is hanging like a flap. This type of wound usually occurs when tissue is forcibly separated or torn from the body. In spite of the severe tissue damage, bleeding is not as bad as might be expected and is relatively easy to control through direct pressure because blood vessels usually constrict and contract at the point of injury.

6. *Amputations.* Amputations are wounds involving the extremities—limbs, hands, feet, fingers, or toes—in which these body parts are completely severed or torn off from the body. A clean-cut amputation may seal off blood vessels and minimize bleeding. A torn amputation, with jagged skin and exposed bones, might bleed profusely.

In 1991, Doug Rheams, a carpenter in Rancho Cordova, California, discovered that even a very severe open wound need not be fatal, or even critically disabling, if appropriate emergency care is given at the scene of the accident.

On the afternoon of September 10, Doug was working, cutting lumber with a power saw at the Redwood Shop, a carpentry shop specializing in custom decks and gazebos. In the office adjoining the workroom, Lori Barudoni, one of the owners of the shop, was doing some paperwork. Lori and Doug were alone in the shop that afternoon, and she came in to ask Doug about his weekend, which he told her had not been a good one—his dog had been run over by a car, and when he went to help the dog, it bit him. Lori went back to the office and became absorbed in her work. Suddenly, the noise of the power saw was punctuated with a loud, terrifying scream. "It was unlike anything I'd ever heard anywhere in my life," Lori said, "and I knew that he'd cut his hand off, even though I wasn't in the same room with him."

She ran into the shop, where Doug was holding his hand and crying in pain as blood spurted from his wrist. She ran back into the office and immediately called 9-1-1. Sacramento County dispatcher Victor Bauthier took the call. "He cut off his hand," Lori yelled into the phone; then, responding to Victor's questioning, gave him the address of the shop. "You've got to get here quick," she added, still yelling excitedly.

"She was a little out of control," said Bauthier. "At times, you have to go in there and bully—tell them 'You need to be calm. We're trying to help the person, and we need you to be calm so we can help him.'"

"Where is he?" Bauthier asked her.

"He's in the workroom."

"Good. Do you have a clean towel? What I want you to do is wrap a towel around his—"

"We don't have any towels," Lori interrupted Bauthier.

"Paper towels? Anything of that nature?" Bauthier asked.

"Nothing—just toilet paper," Lori answered.

"No, that won't do," said Bauthier. "Do you have a T-shirt or anything like that?" he asked, trying to identify something Lori might have on hand that would enable her to put direct pressure on the wound.

"Yes, yes, we have that," she said.

"Good. How bad is the hand? Is it off?" he asked.

"I don't know," Lori answered.

"I want you to wrap it up," Bauthier instructed her.

Lori told Doug to take off his shirt, and wrapped it around his wound.

"What do you want me to do now?" she asked Bauthier, adding, "I think he's gone into shock."

"We want him to lie down," Bauthier answered, articulating each word slowly but forcefully, making certain that Lori both heard and understood.

"Come on, Doug, I want you to lie down—on the ground," she told Rheams, trying to control her panic and worrying that she herself would pass out from the sight of the blood. "I've got to stop the bleeding! I've got to stop the bleeding!" she cried out loud.

"I thought that he had probably ruptured the artery, because of the way the blood was coming out," Bauthier said. "Don't put a tourniquet on it," he told Lori, worried that she would do something that could cause permanent injury. "You don't want to tourniquet things except as a last resort," he explained.

"I've got his shirt on it," she said.

"Just wrap it around," Bauthier said, "and apply pressure."

"Pressure," Lori repeated, following his instructions.

"Apply as much as you can, and don't stop. Now I want you to keep him flat, as he is—"

"Okay."

"—and elevate his legs about 18 inches," Bauthier continued.

"I'm putting them on the bench," Lori said.

"You're doing good work," Bauthier said in encouragement.

"He keeps saying he's going to die," Lori said, agonized.

"No," Bauthier said calmly and reassuringly. "You tell him we're not going to let him do that."

"We're not going to let you do that," Lori said, turning to Doug. "You're just nervous—you're just in shock."

"It's against my rules," Bauthier added jokingly.

"You're not going to die—you're not!" Lori repeated to Doug.

"His eyes kept rolling back in his head, and I would say, 'Come on, Doug, come on,' and his eyes would come back. I knew that if I lost it, there would be no one there to help him," Lori said.

"Does he know how much he cut?" Bauthier asked her.

"How much did you cut, Doug?" she asked Rheams.

"About all the way through," he told her.

"About all the way through," she repeated to Bauthier.

"The hand has not been basically amputated, right?" Bauthier asked, trying to get a clear picture of the injury.

"It's through the bone," Lori said.

"Through the bone—so it's hanging pretty much by the skin?"

"Yes," Laurie said, and then turned all her attention to comforting Doug. "Just think of everybody that's on their way here that's going to take care of you," she told him. "They've got a whole crew coming."

"That a girl—good work," said Bauthier, who could hear her through the phone, encouragingly.

"So just hang on," she told Doug.

"I'm going to die," he said, in agony and panic.

"No, you're not going to die," she said firmly. "We're not going to let that happen."

"Good girl," said Bauthier. "Good girl."

"It's okay," she said to Doug. "It's going to be okay. Let's say a prayer, okay?"

"Okay," Doug responded weakly.

"Oh, dear Lord, please help Doug right now," Lori prayed aloud. "Help him to get through this. Take his hand and walk with him. Give them godspeed on the way here."

"When she started saying that prayer, that was the thing that got to me most on that phone call," Bauthier said.

"Tell the ambulance to hurry," Lori said. And within moments, she and Doug could hear the siren of the rescue unit from the Sacramento County Fire Department. "They're here," she said to Bauthier, hearing the sound in the street. "Can I leave him here?"

"No, no no," he told her. "I want you to hang in along with me until they get to him."

"They're here," she said again, as the rescue team walked through the door.

"Okay," Bauthier said.

"He says it's through the bone," Lori told the rescue team. "He's concerned that he's lost too much blood."

"We're going to take care of him. We're going to take care of him," said one of the team reassuringly.

"When I heard John's voice, I knew she was in good hands," Bauthier said.

"Okay, good-bye," he told Lori.

"Good-bye," she said, relief evident in her voice.

"Looking at the scene, and the amount of blood on the floor and on the wall, I estimated that he had lost 15% of his total blood volume," said one of the rescuers. "With arterial bleeding, a person could die within a few minutes from loss of blood. We virtually constructed a splint from the lower part of his arm all the way up to his fingertips. Doug was very pale. He was telling us that he didn't want to lose his hand. He was telling us that he didn't want to die."

Doug was taken by Lifeflight helicopter to the trauma unit of the University of California Davis Medical Center, where his father, Russ, was waiting for him. "Before they took Doug into surgery, he looked at me and said, 'Well, I guess I'm going to lose my hand.' And I said, "No, no, no, you're not going to lose your hand. Everything's going to be all right. Don't worry about it.' And all the time I was thinking, 'Yes, you are going to lose your hand.'"

Chief orthopedic surgeon and hand specialist David Steinberg performed the operation. "If this had happened 20 or 30 years ago, I think his chances of having a functional hand would have been greatly decreased," Steinberg said. "Technology is now advanced enough that we expect a fair degree of success from this operation." Ten months after Doug's hand had been reattached, he had regained partial use of it, and was anticipating recovery of 90% to 95% of full function, and a return to his carpentry work. Most important, he was grateful to be alive.

"I was real scared that I was going to bleed to death," Doug said. "It's a good thing Lori was there— I really appreciate what she did. I couldn't have made it without her."

"I don't think I did anything extraordinary," Lori said. "I think I did what I was told—and I called 9-1-1. That's the great thing. Once you get hold of them, they'll tell you what to do."

"To me, that's all the gratitude I ever need," said Victor Bauthier. "Just so long as I know that things have worked out and that the help was there for them. That's what my job is all about—helping people."

"You can't be too careful when you're working around equipment like that," Doug said. "No matter how much of a habit you've gotten into of doing the same thing every day, it's still dangerous. You've really got to pay attention to what you're doing and take your time."

"From the very first day, I was teasing him about what a lousy way to get out of working for a living—to try to cut your hand off. But the teasing is all a cover-up so I don't have to think about what I'm really feeling," said Doug's father. "What I'm really feeling is, I could have lost my son."

In cases of severe open wounds, where bleeding is profuse, do not waste time trying to wash the wound. This will be done routinely as part of the care given at the medical facility to which the victim is taken. It is more important to control bleeding and dress the wound as described below. Seek medical care by either calling EMS personnel or transporting the victim to a medical facility. Recommend to the victim that he or she get a tetanus booster shot if he or she has not had one within the last 5 to 10 years.

Treatment for Major Open Wounds:

1. Call EMS personnel.
2. Carefully cut away clothing so that the wound can be seen.
3. If loose foreign particles are around the wound, wipe them away with some clean material, al-

ways wiping *away* from the wound. If possible, do not touch the wound with your hands, clothing, or anything that is not clean. Do *not* waste time trying to wash the wound.

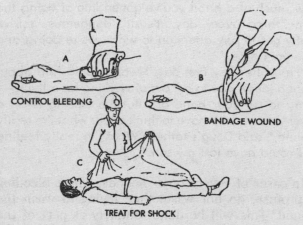

A

CONTROL BLEEDING

B

BANDAGE WOUND

C

TREAT FOR SHOCK

First Aid for Open Wounds

4. Do *not* attempt to remove foreign material that is deeply embedded in muscle or other soft tissue, since this may aggravate bleeding. This must be done by a doctor.
5. Control bleeding by direct pressure and elevation. Apply direct pressure by placing a sterile dressing over the wound. If nothing sterile is available, use any clean covering such as a towel, tie, handkerchief, sock, disposable gloves, or plastic wrap. If no such material is available, have the injured person use his or her hand. As a last resort, use your own bare hand.
6. If the victim has an object impaled in the wound, do *not* remove it. Use bulky dressings

to stabilize it. Any movement of the object can result in further tissue damage. Control bleeding by bandaging the dressings in place around the object.

7. Place a sterile dressing compress or gauze over the wound and bandage in place to maintain pressure on the wound. (*Note:* A dressing is a pad placed directly on the wound to absorb blood and other liquids and to prevent infection. Most are porous to allow air to circulate. A bandage is any material used to wrap or cover any part of the body. It is used to hold dressings in place, maintain pressure to control bleeding, protect a wound from dirt and infection, and provide support for an injured body part.) All dressings should be wide enough to completely cover the wound and the area around it.

8. Protect compresses or gauze dressings with a cover bandage. Triangular and cravat bandages, which can be made from any clean cloth, are made as follows:

1. To make a *triangular bandage,* cut a piece of cloth 36 inches to 40 inches square, and then cut the square in half along the diagonal.

2. Make a medium-width *cravat bandage* as follows:

a. Fold the point of a triangular bandage over to the middle of the base.

b. Keep folding the bandage over until it is the desired width.

Two commonly available commercial bandages are the bandage compress and the roller bandage. A bandage compress is a thick gauze dressing attached to a gauze bandage, which can be tied in place. It is specifically designed to help control severe bleeding and usually comes in a sterile package.

Roller bandages, which are made from gauze or some similar porous material, come in assorted widths and lengths, from ½ inch to 12 inches wide and from 5 to 10 yards long. A roller bandage is usually wrapped around the injured body part, over a dressing, overlapping several times until the dressing is completely covered. It can be tied or taped in place.

9. If blood soaks through the bandage, apply additional dressings and cover with another bandage. Do *not* remove blood-soaked dressings or bandages.

10. Keep the victim quiet and lying still. Any movement will increase circulation, which could restart the bleeding.

11. Calm and reassure the victim.

12. Treat for shock (see p. 305).

Special Treatment for Specific Open Wounds

Puncture wounds: Do not attempt to remove any foreign object deeply embedded in the wound. Encourage bleeding to wash out germs by gently pressing on the sides of the wound.

Amputations: If the victim has an amputation in which a body part has been completely severed, retrieve the severed part and wrap it in sterile gauze, if available, or any clean material such as a handkerchief or washcloth. Place the wrapped part in a plastic bag and, if possible, keep it cool by placing the bag on ice. Make certain that the part is transported to the medical facility with the victim.

INTERNAL BLEEDING

Internal bleeding is the escape of blood from damaged arteries, veins, or capillaries into spaces of the body. Bruising, in which blood from injured capillaries seeps into adjoining tissue and collects visibly beneath the skin, is a minor form of internal bleeding. Severe internal bleeding (usually in the chest or abdominal cavity) generally occurs from the impact of a hard, blunt force, as in automobile accidents or falls from a great height. It can also be the result of certain fractures in which a bone ruptures an organ or a major blood vessel or can be caused by deep penetration by a sharp object, such as a knife, damaging internal structures.

Signs and Symptoms of Internal Bleeding

➤ Discoloration of the skin, pain, swelling, or tenderness where the injury is suspected

➤ Soft tissues, such as abdominal muscle, that is tender, swollen, hard, or in spasm

➤ Bleeding from the mouth, rectum, or other body orifice

➤ Symptoms of shock (due to the body's inability to adjust to the loss of blood):

• Dizziness, especially when going from lying down to standing—this may be the earliest sign of internal bleeding

- Cold, clammy, pale, or bluish skin
- Eyes dull, vision clouded, and pupils enlarged
- Weak, rapid pulse
- Shallow, rapid breathing
- Nausea and vomiting
- Excessive thirst
- Feeling of weakness and helplessness

There is little that you can do to control internal bleeding directly. In severe cases, immediate surgery is necessary, and it is best to call EMS personnel at once. The victim should be kept on his or her side when blood or vomit is coming from his or her mouth. Always consider the possibility of spinal damage when there is a chest injury, and treat the victim accordingly. Maintain an open airway and treat for shock (see p. 305). Never give the victim anything by mouth.

Closed Wounds

Because there is no break in the skin, closed wounds are not always easy to identify. Minor closed wounds, in which only superficial bruising is involved, do not require special medical care. Usually as the result of minor falls or bumps, soft tissues beneath the skin are damaged and small blood vessels ruptured, releasing blood into surrounding tissues. The wound appears red at first, then darkens to blue or purple.

Suspect serious internal damage if the victim has fallen from a height or received a severe body blow to the chest, abdomen, head, or spine. Seek medical care promptly if any of the signs or symptoms listed below are present.

Signs and Symptoms of Internal Injuries:

➤ Pain and tenderness at the site of the injury and redness where the blow occurred
➤ Severe pain or inability to move without pain
➤ Vomit that resembles coffee grounds
➤ Coughed-up blood that is bright red
➤ Stools containing dark, tarry material or bright red blood
➤ Urine containing blood
➤ Pale skin
➤ Cold, clammy skin
➤ Rapid but weak pulse
➤ Rapid breathing
➤ Dizziness
➤ Swelling
➤ Restlessness
➤ Thirst

Treatment to Be Administered While Waiting for EMS Personnel to Arrive:

1. Maintain an open airway and restore breathing if necessary (see p. 160).
2. Keep the victim lying down and quiet.
3. If the victim is vomiting, turn his or her head to the side to prevent choking.
4. If the victim is having difficulty breathing, raise his or her shoulders with a pillow.
5. Check for broken bones and treat accordingly.

6. Keep the victim comfortably warm.
7. Do *not* give the victim anything to eat or drink, including water.
8. Reassure the victim.

A rupture or a hernia is a closed wound resulting from a combination of weaknesses of tissues and muscular strain. The most common form of rupture is a protrusion of an internal organ through the wall of the abdomen, usually occurring just above the groin.

Signs and Symptoms of a Rupture:

> Sharp, stinging pain
> Feeling of something giving way at the site of the rupture
> Swelling
> Possible nausea and vomiting

Treatment for a Rupture or Hernia:

1. Call EMS personnel or transport the injured person to a medical facility while he or she is lying down, with his or her knees drawn up.
2. Do *not* attempt to force the protrusion back into the cavity.
3. Place the victim on his or her back with his or her feet flat on the floor and knees drawn up.
4. Place a blanket or other padding under the victim's knees.

CHEST WOUNDS

Traffic accidents are the most frequent cause of traumatic injuries to the chest, but chest injuries can also be caused by falls, sport accidents, and a variety of crushing or penetrating forces.

Chest wounds may be open or closed. An open wound may be caused by an object puncturing or lacerating the chest from the outside, or by fractured ribs breaking through the skin. Closed wounds are usually caused by a blunt object hitting the chest or a fall.

General Signs and Symptoms of Chest Injuries:

- Difficulty breathing
- Severe pain in the chest, especially at the site of the injury
- Reddened, pale, or bluish discoloration of the skin
- Deformity of the rib cage
- Coughing up blood

Puncture Wound to the Chest

Puncture wounds to the chest can be minor or life threatening. If the puncture is forceful enough to cause a deep, open wound, penetrating the chest cavity or the lung, air can flow in and out of the wound with breathing instead of in and out of the lungs, creating a life-threatening situation. Every time the victim breathes, you hear a sucking sound coming from the wound. Without proper care, the victim's condition will worsen, as the affected lung or lungs fail to function and breathing becomes more difficult. A deep puncture can also injure other structures within the chest and cause varying amounts of internal bleeding.

In August 1992, Patty Richter of Cincinnati, Ohio, discovered how easily a life-threatening puncture wound to the chest can occur when a young child is left unsupervised within reach of a pair of scissors.

"I was giving my 1-year-old, Ryan, a bath in the kitchen sink and talking on the telephone," Patty said, remembering. Meanwhile, her eldest son, Mark, Jr. and his girlfriend, Shanna Rathbone, were in the family room watching television. Four-year old Alex, Patty's middle son, who had become very close to Shanna, came and asked Shanna to help him wash his hands in the bathroom by turning the taps, which were too tight for him to open. "I feel like a member of the family," Shanna said, "and I always have, from the first day I came over. That's just how the Richters are." Shanna walked Alex back to the bathroom, turned on the water for him, and left him to finish the job of washing on his own.

Lying on a shelf, under the small towel that Alex took to dry his hands, were the scissors his mother used to give family members haircuts. Minutes later, he walked into the kitchen, holding the scissors up in front of him, and told his mother, "Mommy, I fell on these."

"I looked at his chest, and there was just a small drop of blood, so I took the washcloth and I dabbed it," Patty said. "Then I screamed." Her scream brought Shanna and Mark running into the kitchen.

"I looked at Alex and I saw this hole in his chest—you could see straight down into his chest. It was just like a great tunnel, going straight down," Shanna said. Patty handed the stricken child to Shanna and called 9-1-1.

Union Township dispatcher Patty Bates was on duty by herself that afternoon. "I heard a very hysterical woman saying that her son had been stabbed and that he had pulled the scissors out himself," Bates said. "I started to worry because I'd always been told that if you're stabbed with something, it's better to leave it in." Rescue units with the Union Township Fire Department were immediately dispatched to the scene.

"I need them to hurry—please tell them to hurry," the distraught mother told Bates, who gave her instructions for immediate first aid. "She told me to apply pressure to the wound," Patty said, "and I hung the phone up. He was just like a limp washrag in your hand, so I was getting more hysterical as the time went on. And then luckily, for some God-given reason, my husband came home."

"I pulled in the driveway, and Mark came up to me and told me Alex had gotten hurt," said Mark, Sr., the boys' father. "I thought, 'We'll take him to the doctor, get stitches, and that will be the end of that.'" Then he went inside and discovered, to his horror, just what the situation was. "What happened?" he asked Patty.

"He fell on my hair-cutting scissors," she said, in tears.

"When I pulled the rag away from Alex's chest, you could actually look inside the chest," Mark said. "He was gray. His lips were blue. The last thing he said to me was 'I'm sleepy.' And that was it."

Among those responding to the emergency call was paramedic Jeff Jackson. "About halfway there," said Jackson, "our dispatcher called us back and advised us that the child was turning blue, which immediately heightened our response. This child has been stabbed, he could be in cardiac arrest, and we're thinking the worst."

"He was getting real listless. I didn't know what to do. You're holding your son and he's dying," Mark said. "There's nothing you're going to be able to do for him." Meanwhile, Patty kept talking to Alex and calling his name, hoping by some miracle that her son would start to respond. Then the anxious family heard the sound of the sirens on the rescue vehicles.

"When the father first came out of the house, I immediately recognized who he was," Jeff Jackson said. "Mark had been in the fire department with me a few years ago, and, ironically, he had left the fire department because he could not deal with injured and sick children. As soon as I looked at the child, I knew he was in a life-threatening situation. He was blue around the lips, blue around the fingertips, which immediately told me that his body was shutting down."

Paramedic Pam Kratzer asked to see the scissors. "The blood on the scissors was 2 inches up on the blades, so we knew that it had punctured at least 2 inches into his body," Kratzer said. "That means they could have not only punctured his lungs and heart, but also gone into his spine."

Jackson realized that Alex needed to have surgery immediately, and asked another EMS technician to check on the availability of an AirCare helicopter to transport the child. "I thought this was this child's only hope," he said.

"Okay, Dad," Kratzer told Mark, gently but insistently, "I need you to hand Alex to me."

"The father did not want to release the child from his arms, and I thought, 'How can I ask this father to lay this child down, knowing that this may be the last time he can hold him?'" she said.

"We need you folks to get right down there to meet us when we get there," Jackson told Alex's parents. "He's going to be fine."

"They kept telling us, 'We need you to leave,'" Patty said. "And I came out of the house thinking that he was dying and they wanted us out of the way. They didn't want us to be there when he died."

Alex was taken to the nearest open field, where he was met by a University of Cincinnati Hospital Air-Care helicopter. The medical team on board included flight nurse Carol Patterson-Downing. "At the time the child was in extreme shock," Patterson-Downing said. "He wasn't breathing well, and his blood pressure was very, very low. The best thing to do was to get him to the operating room at Children's Hospital."

Mark and Patty arrived at the hospital just in time to see Alex briefly before he was wheeled into the operating room. "It was only for few minutes that we got to take a look at him," Mark said. "You want to touch him, you want to talk to him, but you know you can't. I thought that probably would be the last time that I would get to see him."

Alex had been prepared for surgery as soon as he reached the hospital. The operation was performed by surgeon Victor Garcia. "Literally every second mattered," said Dr. Garcia, "because if you have uncontrolled bleeding in the chest, there is an ever-increasing likelihood that the bleeding will result in irreversible consequences that would ultimately kill the child. Once we opened the chest, we found that there was blood inside the sack around the heart. It takes only a small amount of blood in the pericardium to interfere with the ability of the heart to pump." Dr. Garcia operated for 6 hours, repairing the ruptured pericardium. Finally, a nurse came out to the waiting room to tell the Richters that they could see their son.

"They had to cut him from the top of his chest all the way down to his groin area," Patty said. "He had 45 staples down his little, tiny body. He looked pathetic. I wanted to pick him up and kiss his whole face."

"It was as if everybody felt a sigh of relief," said Shanna, who had come to the hospital with the Richters. "Even if he couldn't talk back to us, he was *there*, and in a couple of weeks, he was going to be fine." Eight days later, Alex was released from the hospital.

A year after Alex's accident, he was completely recovered and delighting his family with his energy and enthusiasm for life, but there were lessons they all had learned. "Now I know why when we were kids we were always told by grownups, 'Don't run with scissors,'" Patty said. "If I had any advice to give to people, it would be to make sure that scissors are always put away where children can't get to them."

"Scissors and Dad's tools are objects that we use on an everyday basis and don't think about. We need to think of those as lethal weapons," said Jeff Jackson.

"I'm very proud of my son for coming and telling my wife that he had fallen on the scissors," said Mark. "If he hadn't come to tell her, he could have run out in the yard and died. I thought about being an EMT, but that takes a different breed of people. They saved my son's life. I think those people are great."

"You train all your life to help people," Pam Kratzer said, "and this was one instance where you really did help a child."

"Everything came together," said Jeff Jackson. "It was not a one-person or a one-crew effort. All the years, and all the people we've worked on who have not survived—the bad times, the good times—this makes it all worthwhile."

"When I see him out playing, it's amazing," said Patty. "He's got a scar, but that's okay—that's a battle scar to him. He shows it to everybody."

"This is where the doctor cut me," says Alex, raising his shirt. "I won't play with scissors again, because they could hurt you."

"I almost lost him," said Patty. "And that's probably why he's pretty spoiled right now. I can't imagine my life without Alex—I just can't imagine it."

Treatment for Severe Puncture Wounds to the Chest:

1. Call EMS personnel.
2. Do *not* remove any object remaining in the wound, as very serious bleeding or other internal life-threatening injuries may result.
3. Immediately cover the entire wound with a dressing that does not allow air to pass through it. Plastic wrap, a plastic bag, or aluminum foil folded several times are excellent for this. If none of these materials is available, use dry, sterile gauze, or a clean cloth or clothing. Tape the dressing in place, except for one loose corner, which will allow air to escape during exhalation. If no dressing is available, place a hand on each side of the wound and firmly push the skin together to close the wound. Apply an airtight ban-

dage over the wound and fasten with tape, if available.

4. Maintain an open airway and restore breathing if necessary (see p. 160).

5. Treat for shock. You may have to raise the victim's shoulders slightly to assist breathing (see pp. 305–06).

6. Do *not* give the victim anything to eat or drink, as this may cause choking.

ABDOMINAL WOUNDS

The abdomen is the area of the body just below the chest and above the pelvis. The area is easily injured because it is not surrounded by bones. The vital organs the abdomen contains, chief among which are the liver, the spleen, and the stomach, tend to bleed profusely when damaged.

Wounds of the abdomen can be open or closed, and even with a closed wound, the rupture of an organ can cause several internal bleeding, resulting in shock. Abdominal wounds are often extremely painful, and serious reactions can occur when organs leak blood or other substances into the abdomen.

Signs and Symptoms of Abdominal Injury:

➤ Extreme pain
➤ Bruising of the area
➤ External bleeding
➤ Nausea
➤ Vomiting, with the vomit sometimes containing blood
➤ Weakness

➤ Thirst
➤ Pain, tenderness, or a sensation of tightness in the abdomen
➤ Organs protruding from the abdomen

Treatment for Abdominal Wounds:

1. Call EMS personnel.
2. Maintain an open airway and restore breathing if necessary (see p. 160).
3. Lay the victim carefully on his or her back.
4. Bend the victim's legs at the knees and place a pillow, a rolled towel, a blanket, or clothing under the knees to relax the abdominal muscles.
5. Control bleeding if necessary by direct pressure, but do *not* push organs back inside the abdomen.
6. Remove any clothing from around the wound.
7. Apply sterile dressings loosely over the wound.
8. Cover the entire wound loosely with plastic wrap, if available, or with a sterile pad, clean cloth, clothing, aluminum foil, or similar material.
9. Cover the dressings with a folded towel to maintain warmth.
10. Treat for shock (see p. 305).

PELVIC WOUNDS

The pelvis, which is the lower part of the trunk, contains the bladder, the reproductive organs, and part of the large intestine. Major arteries and nerves pass through it as well. These structures may be damaged by being struck with forceful blows with blunt or penetrating objects or by fractured bones puncturing or lacerating them. The signs and symptoms of pelvic injury are the same as those of abdominal injury. There may also be a loss of sensation in the legs or an inability to move them, which may indicate an injury of the lower spine.

Treatment for Pelvic Wounds:
In general, the treatment is similar to that for abdominal injuries.

1. Try to keep the victim lying down, and do not move him or her if you suspect a spinal injury.
2. Control any external bleeding and cover any protruding organs.
3. Call EMS personnel and treat for shock (see p. 305).
4. If there is an injury to the genitals, it may be extremely painful. Treat any closed wound here as you would any other closed wound. If the wound is open, apply direct pressure with your hand or the victim's hand. If any parts are amputated, wrap them appropriately and make certain they are transported with the victim.

Burns

A burn is an injury to the soft tissue of the body (skin, fat, nerves, or muscles) caused by heat, electricity, chemicals, or radiation. Heat burns, caused by direct contact with fire, hot surfaces, or hot liquids, are the most common burns occurring in the home.

The severity of a burn depends upon the temperature of the heat source, how long exposure is, where on the body the burn is located, how large the burn is, and the age and medical condition of the burn victim. Older people, especially over 60, usually have thinner skins and thus may burn more severely, and children under 5 are especially vulnerable for the same reason. People with chronic medical conditions, particularly those involving the heart or kidneys, also tend to have greater complications from burn wounds.

Amy Rabinovitz and Kelly Unger are mothers who learned through devastating experience the danger of burns to young children, and the importance of following child safety rules.

On a peaceful June afternoon in 1993 in the small town of Hingham, Massachusetts, Amy Rabinovitz was boiling meat in her kitchen while her three children sat in the living room, absorbed in a television program. The baby gate that kept her 14-month-old toddler, Abigail, safely out of the kitchen while Amy was working there had broken, so before touching the pot, Amy looked around to assure herself that she was alone in the room. Seeing that she was, and hearing the comforting sound of the television set and the children's responsive laughter, she proceeded to remove the meat and then turned to pour the hot water and grease down the drain in the sink. To her horror, she found herself tripping over Abigail, who had quickly and silently crawled into the room while her back was turned. The searing liquids spilled down onto the baby's front.

"I grabbed her and the skin peeled off in my hand," Amy said. "I thought I was going to lose her." In spite of her panic, Amy carried Abigail to the shower and doused her with cool water to stop the burning, removed her clothing, and wrapped her in a clean wet towel, as her son, Benjamin, made the critical phone call for help.

Although there is no 9-1-1 system in Hingham, Benjamin was able to reach the fire department quickly because Amy had entered the number in her phone's speed-dial system a month before. He gave them the necessary information, and EMS personnel were there in 3 minutes. One of them was particularly worried, because he realized from the address that Amy was someone he had known since childhood.

"When I first arrived, 40% of the body was burned,

and that's such an insult to the body, just because of the infection alone, that I feared for the baby's life," he said.

Abigail was put on a stretcher to be transported to Southshore Hospital, and Amy observed with terror that her daughter suddenly stopped crying and didn't move. "I thought she had stopped breathing. I thought she had lost it. I thought she was gone."

One of the EMTs started tapping on the bottom of Abigail's feet and calling out her name. "Then she started crying again. The wailing was tough to hear, but I knew that she was breathing," he said.

Because of the seriousness of her condition, Abigail was taken from Southshore to the Shriner's Burns Institute in Boston, where she was treated by Dr. Robert Sheridan. "The liquid poured down from above and the burns were on her face, neck, and shoulders. One third of her skin was gone," Dr. Sheridan said. "In many parts of the world, an injury of this kind to a child this age is lethal. The majority of the burns that we see at the Shriner's are from cooking accidents or bathing accidents. Seventy percent of the burns we treat are from hot liquids."

"I was very surprised at the damage hot water can do. I had always thought that a fire burn or an electrical burn could do a lot more damage," Abigail's father later said.

Abigail was treated at Shriner's for a month, and her parents visited her every day, sharing her agony and her hope. "There's nothing that can prepare you for walking into a burn trauma unit," Abigail's father said. "The first thing that hits you is the smell."

One of the most frustrating things for Abigail's parents was that they could not comfort their child by holding her in their arms. "To see her bandaged up like that, that wasn't my baby. That was somebody else's baby, I kept thinking," said Amy. "The guilt that hits you is incredible. You had to wear rubber gloves and a mask and a plastic apron just to reach through the curtain and touch her. You couldn't just pick up your child and hold her."

"That was one of those little joys that you just don't think about until you lose it for a while," Abigail's father said.

Dressing changes for Abigail's burns were painful events that occurred twice a day. "I cried every time the dressings were changed," Amy said, "and I was there every time."

Abigail's skin graft operations went well, but she contracted pneumonia while in the hospital, which was quickly treated. She was released after a month in the hospital, and returned home to delight her family with her spirit and her energy.

Before Abigail came home from the hospital, the Rabinovitzes bought a new baby gate, "which we use all day and every day," Amy says. "And we always tell the kids, 'Call the ambulance if you think you need it. Don't hesitate.'"

"Because the injury was so severe," her father said, "we didn't think she was going to make it. So just to have that little person running around in the front yard is unbelievably rewarding. We've had some tough times, but it helped to restore a lot of our faith in humanity to know that people, like the people who took care of Abigail, really do care."

 On the morning of December 27, 1991, 5-year-old Megan Unger and her 9-year-old sister, Janet, were watching TV while their mother, Kelly, was taking a shower upstairs. Although she was not allowed to use the stove, Megan, who had watched Kelly making breakfast many times, decided to cook herself some oatmeal.

Standing on a chair, which she pushed next to the stove, to boil the water, she reached across the stove for a wooden spoon with which to stir in the oatmeal. The sleeve of her nightgown touched the flame of the gas burner and ignited, sending fire racing up her arm. Her anguished screams brought Janet racing into the kitchen.

Janet remembered the lesson of "stop, drop, and roll," which she had learned in school. She pulled her hysterical sister off the chair, threw her to the ground, and rolled her over and over to extinguish the flames, then threw a glass of water on her.

Kelly, hearing Megan's screams, raced downstairs, where she found her lying on the floor, severely burned, with her nightgown in tatters. She scooped her wounded daughter up in her arms, ran upstairs to the bathroom, wrapped her in a clean sheet and submerged her in a tub of cool water. Then she called 9-1-1.

"I couldn't believe this was happening to my daughter," Kelly said. "You have children, and they have these perfect bodies. You can't imagine this kind of destruction."

"I knew I had to save my sister," Janet Unger later said. "Stop, drop, and roll. Megan didn't know because she was just in kindergarten, so I had to do it."

"I'm grateful for Janet," Kelly said. "If Janet hadn't been there, Megan might not be with us today."

Firefighters and paramedics from the Valley Vista Fire Department arrived, assessed the seriousness of the situation, and decided that helicopter transport was required. Megan was driven in an ambulance to a nearby field and then flown to the San Bernadino County Medical Center, where she was diagnosed as having second-degree and third-degree burns over 30% of her body. Megan was in the hospital for 5½ weeks, during which time she had three skin graft surgeries.

"I never knew how serious burns were until this happened," said her father. "I never looked at it as a life-threatening event. Now we're facing months of therapy and years of skin grafts. But even though she's scarred on the outside, I don't believe she's going to be scarred on the inside, and that's where the true beauty is."

General Rules for Treating Burns

Treatment for burns should be directed at relieving pain, excluding air from the injured area, preventing infection, and preventing or alleviating shock.

Tissue will continue to burn for minutes after the heat source is removed, so cooling the burned area to prevent further tissue damage is important. Large amounts of cool or tepid water are best for this purpose, although anything cool and drinkable, such as soda or a milkshake, can be applied to the burned area if water is not readily available. Ice or ice water should never be used, because they can cause critical body heat loss.

Plenty of time should be allowed for the cooling process to take place. So long as pain continues or the edges of the burned area feel warm to the touch, cooling by immersion in cool or tepid water or the application of wet, cool—but not cold—compresses should continue.

Once the area is cool, remove clothing from the burn site by gently pulling or cutting it away. Do not try to remove any clothing that is stuck to the skin. Except for the burned area, the injured person should be kept covered because there is a tendency to chill.

Cover the burned area with a clean, sterile, non-fluffy dressing, and bandage loosely, so no pressure is put on the wound. This will help prevent infection and protect sensitive nerve endings, which may be exposed. Do *not* apply butter, oils, or ointments. These will only seal in the heat. Bandage so that burned surfaces are not in contact with each other, such as those between fingers and toes, the ears and the side of the head, the undersurface of the arm and the chest wall, the folds of the groin, and similar places.

Classification and Treatment of Specific Burns

Burns are generally classified by their depth, or how many layers of tissue are affected. All burns should be evaluated by a physician.

A *superficial, minor, or first-degree burn* affects only the top layer of skin, which becomes painful, slightly reddened, and sometimes swollen. Such burns, in which no blistering occurs, are frequently caused by sunburn or brief exposure to hot objects, hot water, or steam.

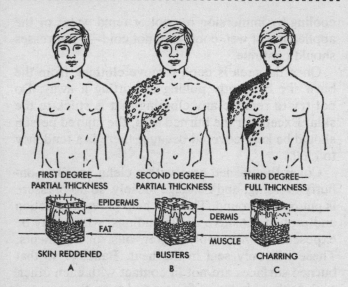

FIRST DEGREE—
PARTIAL THICKNESS

SECOND DEGREE—
PARTIAL THICKNESS

THIRD DEGREE—
FULL THICKNESS

EPIDERMIS

DERMIS

FAT

MUSCLE

SKIN REDDENED
A

BLISTERS
B

CHARRING
C

Classification of Burns by Degree of Injury

Treatment for a First-Degree Burn:

1. Immediately put the burned area under cool or tepid running water, or apply a cool-water compress (towel, washcloth, or clean handkerchief soaked in cool—but not cold—water) until the pain subsides.
2. Apply a clean, nonfluffy bandage to the burned area.

First-degree burns generally heal in 5 to 6 days without permanent scarring.

Partial-thickness, moderate, or second-degree burns affect both the top layer (epidermis) and the underlayer (dermis) of the skin. These burns are most frequently caused by deep sunburn, hot liquids, and flash burns from gasoline and other substances. The burned area is reddened, blotchy or streaky, painful, usually blistered, and often swollen. The swelling may last for several days. The blisters may break and release a clear fluid, and the subsequently exposed tissue may have a wet, shiny appearance.

Treatment for a Second-Degree Burn:

1. Flush the burned area with cool or tepid water or apply cool—but not cold—water compresses until the pain subsides and the edges of the area are no longer warm to the touch.
2. Using a clean towel or other soft material, carefully pat the area dry.
3. Loosely bandage the burned area with a dry, nonfluffy, sterile dressing or clean cloth.
4. Elevate burned arms or legs higher than the victim's heart.
5. Seek medical attention.

Do *not* break blisters intentionally.

Warning: Second-degree burns of the face, hands or feet, or genitalia or those covering more than 15% of the body of an adult or more than 10% of the body of a child or a person over 55 require *prompt medical attention*. Body surface can be estimated by calculating that the hand, including the fingers, represents about 1% of the total area.

Second-degree burns usually heal within 3 to 4 weeks, and some scarring may occur.

Full-thickness, critical, or third-degree burns destroy both layers of the skin and destroy or seriously damage underlying tissue including fat, muscle, nerve, and bone. These burns are generally caused by fire or prolonged contact with hot substances, or are electrical burns. The burned area will appear charred (brown or black), with the exposed underlying tissue showing a gray or white color. It may be extremely painful or relatively without sensation if the nerve endings in the skin have been destroyed.

Third-degree burns are considered life-threatening, even when covering a relatively small area of the body. Because of the open nature of the wound, the body quickly loses fluid and shock can occur. They also make the body extremely vulnerable to infection.

Treatment for a Third-Degree Burn:

1. Call an ambulance, remove the victim to the hospital, or contact EMS immediately.
2. If the victim is on fire, smother the flames with a bedspread, rug, jacket, or coat. If these are not available, throw the victim to the ground and roll him or her around the vertical axis of the body until the flames are extinguished.
3. Breathing difficulties may occur with critical burns, especially if they are around the face, neck, and mouth and/or smoke inhalation has occurred. Check to make sure that the victim is still breathing.
4. Cool burns on face, hands, or feet with cool or tepid water or cool—but not cold—compresses.

Do not put cool liquids on large burned areas, because this will result in chilling.

5. Cover the burned area with thick, sterile, non-fluffy dressings. A clean sheet, pillowcase, or disposable diaper can be used for this purpose.

6. While waiting for medical assistance to arrive:

   • Elevate burned hands, arms, legs, or feet higher than the victim's heart.
   • If burns are on head, face, or neck, prop up the victim with pillows. Continue to check to ensure that the victim is still breathing easily. Keep an open airway (see p. 160) if breathing becomes difficult.
   • Treat for shock (see p. 305).

Third-degree burns usually result in scarring. Physical therapy and skin grafts may be required.

Chemical burns can be caused by cleaning solutions, such as household bleach, drain cleaners, toilet-bowl cleaners, paint strippers, and lawn or garden chemicals. The caustic chemicals in these products are usually either strong acids or strong alkalies, which can quickly injure the skin and will continue to do so as long as there is contact.

Treatment for Chemical Burns:

1. If the burn is from a dry chemical, brush it off with a cloth or brush before irrigating the area. Flush the burned area with large quantities of cool, running water for at least 5 minutes and call EMS personnel. Speed and quantity of water are critical in minimizing damage; a tub, buckets

of water, a shower, or a garden hose may be used. Do *not* use a hose at full force, as this may further injure damaged tissue.

2. Keep flushing the burn with water and have the victim remove contaminated clothes while waiting for EMS personnel to arrive.

3. After flushing the burn, follow instructions on the label of the product that caused the burn, if available.

Burn Prevention and Fire Safety

- If your clothes catch fire, do not run. This will simply fan the flames. Instead, "stop, drop, and roll": stop where you are, drop to the ground, and cover your face with your hands and roll over and over to smother the flames.

- Do not run into a burning building to rescue a victim trapped in a fire. You could become a victim yourself.

- If you must escape a fire, crawl on the floor where the air is cooler and cleaner. Smoke inhalation accounts for the majority of fire deaths.

- If you are trapped in a fire, feel a door for heat before opening it. If the door is hot, do not open it. Seek an alternative escape if possible.

- Practice fire drills with your family so that everyone knows what to do in case of a fire. Everyone should have and practice, at least twice a year, a home escape plan that includes knowing two ways out of every room and a meeting place outside. Teach your children that they cannot hide from a fire and that if a fire breaks out in your home, they should always get out of the house, assuming it is safe to do so. If you live in an apartment building with elevators, plan an escape route using the stairs in case of fire.

- If you install bars on your windows to keep out intruders, make sure they have a quick release from the inside so that you can escape in the event of a fire.
- Install smoke detectors in your house, check them weekly, and replace batteries with fresh ones at least once a year. For further protection, consider installing an automatic sprinkler system.
- Find out from your local fire department about the four classes of fire extinguishers, and how they should be used. Get the one that is most appropriate for your home. Learn how to use it and keep it out of the reach of children.
- Buy flame-retardant furniture, rugs, curtains, drapes, and bedding, especially for children's rooms. Buy sleepwear for children made from flame-retardant material and do not allow them to sleep in underwear or playwear that is not flame retardant.
- Check and inspect your electric blanket each year before using it.
- Sleeping with the bedroom doors closed may help protect you if fire breaks out in your home.
- Cold-weather months are the peak period for home fires owing to the increased use of heating equipment. Never leave portable heaters or space heaters operating unattended. Turn them off before leaving the room or going to sleep.

(Only wood-burning stoves specifically designed to burn overnight should be left on while sleeping.) When using a portable heater in the home, make sure that it is far enough away from the wall, the bed, curtains, and anything else that might be combustible to keep them from igniting.

- If you must use extension cords, make certain that they can carry the amount of current you need, and do not use them for long periods of time. They are designed only for temporary use and can crack or wear if used too long, causing a fire hazard. Do not use an extension cord for a major heat-producing appliance. Never cover any electrical cord with a rug or other object. Do not overload any one extension cord or electrical outlet.

- Short circuits can cause fires. A fuse that blows repeatedly or a circuit breaker that trips repeatedly may signal a problem.

- Keep household appliances unplugged when not in use.

- In a severe thunderstorm, unplug the television and other major appliances. Electrically charged appliances present a potential fire hazard.

- Position heat-producing electrical appliances such as toasters, microwaves, televisions, and stereo and video equipment so they have ample air space around and under them to prevent overheating.

- If you have a fireplace, make sure it is well screened and that the fire is completely extinguished before you go to bed.

- Have your chimney swept periodically.
- More people in the United States die from the careless disposal of smoking materials than from any other type of fire. *Never* smoke in bed. Use deep, sturdy ashtrays; douse butts with water before discarding; and check behind and under furniture cushions before leaving home or going to sleep to make sure no butts are smoldering.
- To prevent accidental scalding, turn your water heater down to 120° Fahrenheit.
- Always clean the lint from inside and around the dryer after every dryer cycle. Never leave the house with the dryer running.
- Never leave cooking equipment operating unattended. It is the leading cause of home fires in the United States.
- Never hang anything flammable above the stove and don't wear clothes with loose sleeves while cooking.
- Do not put anything on top of your stove except cookware.
- Turn handles of pots and pans to the rear of the stove.
- Do not store food, snacks, toys, or other things appealing to children above the stove.
- Keep baking soda, flour, a pot lid, or salt on hand to snuff out small pan fires.
- If something in your oven catches fire, close the oven door to suffocate the flames and turn off the oven. If something in your microwave is on fire, keep the door closed until the fire goes out. An open door will allow air to rush in and fuel the fire.

- To keep children from burning themselves, cover stove knobs with safety covers or remove them entirely when not in use.
- Keep all hot liquids and food out of children's reach.
- Do not use tablecloths around children. They can pull a tablecloth, causing hot foods or liquids to spill on them.
- Use your barbecue in an open area. Do not use lighter fluid, which can flare suddenly. Douse all the embers when you're finished.
- Do not use gasoline to build a fire.
- Store flammable liquids, such as gasoline, lighter fluid, and paint thinner outside your home in a safe place, out of the reach of children. Put them where they will not overheat and will not come into contact with a heat source.
- Teach your children not to start fires and to give all matches and cigarette lighters to adults when they find them. Keep matches and lighters out of the reach of children.
- Never cover a lamp shade with a cloth or paper.
- Teach your children, even preschoolers, the basic principles of fire safety, and be certain that your children's babysitter knows them. About 80% of all U.S. fire deaths occur in the home.

Holiday Fire Safety:

- Do not place your Christmas tree near any heat sources.

- Use only tested and approved electrical lights on your Christmas tree, and don't overload the outlets.
- Do not leave Christmas lights on overnight.
- Do not use lighted candles on Christmas trees or evergreen decorations.

Choking

Choking occurs when the airway is fully or partially blocked by some foreign object, such as a piece of food, chewing gum, tobacco, a small toy, or fluids like vomit, blood, mucus, or saliva, causing unconsciousness or respiratory arrest. When a person tries to breathe and swallow at the same time, contrary signals are sent to the epiglottis, the flap of skin that normally covers the trachea during swallowing and covers the esophagus during inhalation. Consequently, it may leave the trachea open at the wrong moment, allowing a foreign object to enter. Obstruction by a foreign object can occur during eating from attempting to swallow a large piece of poorly chewed food, meat being the most common food with which this happens.

This can happen more easily when alcohol is drunk before or during meals, since alcohol dulls the nerves that aid swallowing. Wearing dentures can also make choking more likely because they make it difficult to know whether food is thoroughly chewed before swallowing. Eating quickly and talking or laughing with your mouth full can be other contributing causes, as can walking, playing, or running with food or anything else in the mouth.

Grabbing the throat with one or both hands is the universal distress signal for choking, and it occurs involuntarily when the airway is fully blocked. If the airway is fully blocked, the victim will be unable to speak, breathe, or cough and may turn pale white, gray, or blue. If the airway is partially blocked, the victim may begin gasping or breathing noisily. Partial blockage can easily turn into full blockage, and both must be recognized and treated immediately, or unconsciousness due to lack of oxygen, followed by death, can quickly occur.

David Cooper of Salcedo, Missouri, had been involved in EMS for 15 years, but never realized the importance of instructing young children in emergency first aid for choking until one evening in March 1992, when he left his 8-year-old son Michael and his 11-year-old daughter Mary Beth in the care of their 73-year-old great-grandmother, Mary Cantrell.

This was a biweekly event for David, who brought his children to his grandmother's house, where they all had dinner together before he left to attend a class. "My grandmother fixed us fried chicken with all the trimmings," David said. "She's always been an excellent cook. It was just like any of the other nights. When the meal was over, I got up and did my routine with the kids—giving them their hugs and kisses and wishing everybody good-bye."

"I helped my grandma with the dishes for a little while," Mary Beth said. Then she went into the living room to join her brother in front of the television set.

After a little while, "we heard my grandmother banging on the kitchen counter. We went into the kitchen, and when she turned around, her face was real blue."

Finding a piece of unfinished chicken on her plate, Mrs. Cantrell had decided to eat it before loading the plate into the dishwasher. Hastily pushing it into her mouth, she managed to lodge it in her throat and, gasping for air but unable to speak, banged on the counter to get the children's attention.

"I knew I had to do *something*, and Mary Beth said, 'Dial 9-1-1,'" Michael said.

"She was holding onto the counter and trying to get her breath, but she just couldn't. I was afraid she was going to die. I saw people on 'Rescue 911' doing the Heimlich maneuver and I just thought that's what needed to be done to my grandma," Mary Beth said. She proceeded to wrap her arms around her great-grandmother's waist and give two upward thrusts, but with no results. Michael reported getting a busy signal on the 9-1-1 line, and they traded places, with Mary Beth taking the phone and Michael performing the Heimlich maneuver on Mrs. Cantrell.

Mary Beth got through to a dispatcher, but hung up the phone before she could speak and raced across the street to get a neighbor.

"I was so scared that she was going to die," Michael said. "I just wrapped my arms around her and kept pulling." On the fifth thrust, he was successful. "It just flew right out into the sink," Michael said of the piece of chicken that had almost ended his great-grandmother's life.

"I was proud of what they had done," David Cooper said, "and I was surprised, because Michael and Mary Beth had never been trained in the Heimlich maneuver. And when I asked them about it, they promptly informed me that what they had seen they had picked up off 'Rescue 911.'" Nonetheless, nothing can substitute for actual classroom training, where you can understand the do's and the don'ts of providing first aid.

"Before this, I had always believed that instructing young children in emergency first aid was not a good idea. But after seeing what Michael and Mary Beth had done, my attitude changed. I think that a child is capable of picking up and learning anything that you can present to him."

"I'm just so proud that words can't tell it," said Mary Cantrell. "Unless somebody's saved your life, you don't know how to express this."

"My grandma could be gone right now," Mary Beth said, "but she's still with us. And if my brother hadn't done that, she probably wouldn't be."

The goal in all cases for treatment of choking is to fully open the airway as quickly as possible. If the airway is only partially blocked and there is enough air exchange for the victim to cough, he or she should be encouraged to keep coughing to clear the obstruction. If coughing continues without relief, call EMS personnel for assistance. If the airway is fully blocked, abdominal thrusts, also known as the Heimlich maneuver, are the method of choice for opening it.

All choking victims should have a medical examination after the incident, since complications can occur not only from choking, but also from first-aid measures.

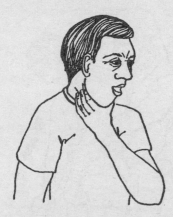

Universal Distress Signal for Choking

Treatment for a Conscious Choking Victim:

1. Without squeezing the victim (who can be sitting or standing), stand behind him or her and put your arms around his or her waist.
2. Make a fist with one hand, with the thumb side against the middle of the victim's abdomen, just above the navel and well below the rib cage.
3. Grasp the fist with the other hand, and give quick upward thrusts, pressing your fist into the victim's abdominal area. This increases the pressure in the abdomen, which pushes up the diaphragm. The increased air pressure in the lungs stimulates coughing, which will often push the foreign object out of the windpipe.
4. The thrusts should be repeated until the object is dislodged or the person becomes unconscious.
5. If the victim is pregnant or too obese for your

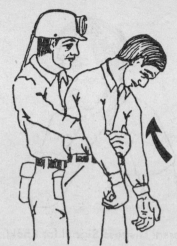

**Abdominal Thrust (Heimlich Maneuver)
with Victim Standing**

arms to reach around his or her waist, use a chest thrust, sliding your arms under the victim's armpits so that you encircle the chest.

6. Make a fist with one hand, placing the thumb side against the center of the victim's sternum (breastbone). Make certain that the fist is not too far down on the sternum, and not on the ribs. The correct position is about two or three finger widths above the lower tip of the sternum.

7. Grab the fist with your other hand and give four quick backward thrusts.

8. If this does not work, stand behind the victim and put one arm around him or her to support the chest with your hand. With your other hand, give four quick blows to the back between the victim's shoulder blades.

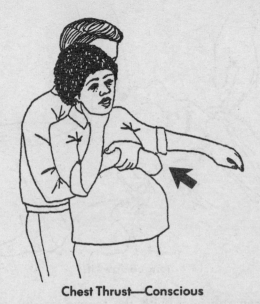

Chest Thrust—Conscious

9. If this does not work, repeat the chest thrusts until the object is expelled or the victim becomes unconscious.

Treatment for a Conscious Choking Victim Who Becomes Unconscious:

If abdominal thrusts do not succeed in removing the obstruction, the victim will eventually become unconscious. When this happens:

1. Lay the victim on the floor on his or her back and call EMS personnel.

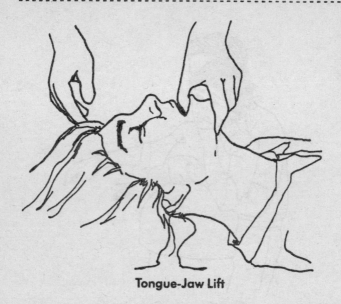

Tongue-Jaw Lift

2. Open the jaws with the tongue-jaw lift or the cross-finger technique, and attempt to manually remove the foreign object with a finger sweep.

   • *Tongue-jaw lift:* Open the victim's mouth by grasping both the tongue and the lower jaw and lifting both together.
   • *Cross-finger technique:* Cross your thumb under your index finger. Brace your thumb and finger against the victim's upper and lower teeth and push your fingers apart to separate the jaws.
   • *Finger sweep:* Lifting the lower jaw with one hand, insert the index finger of the other hand down the inside of the cheek and into the throat to the base of the tongue. Use a hooklike mo-

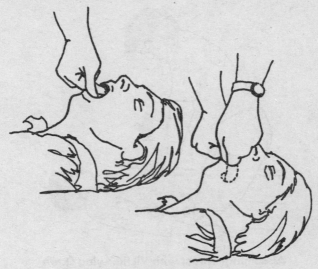

Cross-Finger Technique

tion, sweeping the finger across the back of the throat, to dislodge the obstruction. Be careful not to push the object farther into the airway.

3. Attempt to open the victim's airway using the head-tilt/chin-lift method and give two slow rescue breaths (see p. 161.) Often, when someone is unconscious, the person's throat muscles will relax sufficiently to permit air to get past the obstruction into the lungs.

4. If the chest does not appear to rise with the breaths, assume that the airway is still obstructed, and give five abdominal thrusts. To give abdominal thrusts when the victim is lying

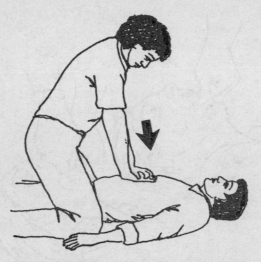

Abdominal Thrust with Victim Lying Down

down, straddle the victim's hips or, if this is not possible, one of his or her legs. Put the heel of one of your hands on the middle of the victim's abdomen, between the rib cage and the navel, with the fingers pointing toward the victim's head. Place your other hand over the first, also pointing the fingers toward the head. Move your shoulders directly over the victim's abdomen and give 6 to 10 quick upward thrusts into the abdominal area.

5. Repeat steps 2 and 3 (opening the mouth, finger sweep, and rescue breathing) and, if you are still unable to get breath into the victim's lungs, repeat the thrusts. Continue repeating this sequence of thrusts, finger sweep, and rescue

breaths until the obstruction is cleared, you can breathe into the victim, or EMS personnel arrive. If your first few attempts to clear the airway are not successful, *do not stop*. The longer the victim is without oxygen, the more the muscles of the throat will relax, increasing the possibility that you will be able to clear the obstruction.

Treatment for an Unconscious Choking Victim:

1. Position the victim on his or her back, on a rigid surface.
2. If the victim is not breathing, start with the head-tilt/chin-lift and give two slow rescue breaths (see p. 161).
3. If the breaths do not go in, you may not have

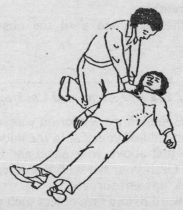

Chest Thrust with Victim Lying Down

tilted the victim's head far enough to release the tongue, so retilt the head and repeat the breaths.

4. If the chest still does not rise, assume that the airway is obstructed by some foreign object or substance. Follow steps 4 and 5 above.

5. If chest thrusts are required because the victim is pregnant or obese, kneel to one side of the victim so you can easily reach his or her chest.

6. Put the heel of one hand on the lower half of the sternum, approximately 1 to 1½ inches above the tip, with the fingers elevated and pointing horizontally across the body. Place the other hand on top of and parallel to the first. Lean over so that your shoulders are directly over your hands, lock your elbows, and do 6 to 10 quick downward thrusts, each one compressing the chest from 1½ to 2 inches.

7. Open the mouth using one of the methods described above, do the finger sweep, and give two rescue breaths.

8. Repeat the sequence until the obstruction is cleared.

Treatment If You Are Alone and Choking:

1. Use the Heimlich maneuver on yourself, placing the thumb side of your fist in the middle of your abdomen just above your navel and below your rib cage. Grab your fist with the other hand and give quick upward thrusts.

2. Bend forward over a firm object such as the back of a chair, a railing, or a sink to exert pressure

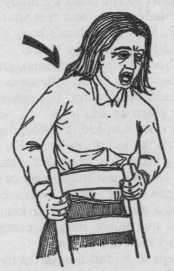

Abdominal Thrust Using a Chair

on your abdomen. Do *not* use an object with a sharp edge or a corner on which you might injure yourself.

Treatment for Choking If the Victim Is an Infant (First Year After Birth):

1. If an infant cannot cough, cry, or breathe; is coughing weakly; or is making high-pitched noises, assume that he or she is choking and call EMS for help.
2. Supporting the infant's head and neck, turn the infant face down on your forearm.

3. Give support to the head by firmly holding the jaw from underneath, and rest your forearm on your thigh, with the infant's body tilted so that the head is lower than the trunk.

4. With the heel of your other hand, give five back blows between the infant's shoulder blades. The blows should be forceful, but more gentle than the blows given an adult.

5. If this does not succeed is dislodging the foreign object, turn the infant on his or her back firmly supporting his or her head and neck.

6. Place the second and third finger of one of your hands on the infant's breastbone, about a finger width below an imaginary line joining the nipples. Give five quick thrusts, compressing the chest ½ to 1 inch each time.

7. Repeat steps 4, 5, and 6 until the foreign object is coughed up or the infant starts to cough, cry, or breathe.

Treatment for Choking If the Infant Becomes Unconscious:

1. Place the infant on a flat, rigid surface.

2. Try to locate and remove the object from the infant's throat. Use the tongue-jaw lift (grasp tongue and lower jaw and lift jaw) to open the mouth, and if the object can be seen, try to remove it with a finger sweep (see pp. 92–93).

3. Open the airway by tilting the head back gently and lifting the chin.

4. Give two rescue breaths: keeping the head tilted back, make a seal around the infant's nose and

mouth with your lips and give two breaths of about 1½ seconds each.

5. If the breaths do not go in (the chest does not rise), put the infant face down on your forearm again and give five back blows.

6. Supporting the head and neck, turn the infant on his or her back, and, resting your forearm on your knee, give five chest thrusts.

7. Repeat steps 1 through 6 until the airway is cleared and the infant starts to breathe or EMS personnel arrive.

Treatment for Choking If the Victim is a Child:

1. Call EMS.

2. Stand or kneel behind the child with your arms around his or her waist.

3. Make a fist with one hand and place the thumb side of the fist against the child's stomach, just above the navel and below the ribs and breastbone.

4. Grab the fist with the other hand and give four quick upward thrusts into the abdomen. Repeat until the object is dislodged or the child begins to cough or breathe.

Treatment for Choking If the Child Becomes Unconscious:

1. Lower the child to the floor and lay him or her on his or her back, face up.

2. Try to locate and remove the object in the child's throat. Open the mouth using the tongue-jaw lift.

If the object is visible, use the finger sweep (see pp. 92–93) to remove it.

3. Open the airway by tilting the head back gently and lifting the chin.

4. Give two rescue breaths. Keeping the head tilted back, pinch the nostrils shut and make a tight seal around the child's mouth with your lips. Give two breaths of about 1½ seconds each.

5. If the air won't go in, give up to five abdominal thrusts. Straddling the child's legs with your knees, place the heel of one hand on his or her abdomen, with your fingers facing up toward his or her head. Place your other hand over and parallel to the first and press in with quick upward thrusts.

6. Repeat steps 2 through 5 until the airway is cleared or EMS personnel arrive.

Tips to Prevent Choking:

- Keep small items such as coins, buttons, and hard candy out of the reach of children and pets.
- Inspect stuffed animals for facial features such as buttons, glass eyes, and other items that can be pulled off and cause a choking hazard.
- Be aware that the most common foods that cause choking in children are hot dogs, hard candy, nuts, popcorn, raw carrots, and peanut butter.
- Never tie a pacifier around a baby's neck.
- Learn how to perform the Heimlich maneuver on adults, children, and infants.

Cold Emergencies

The human body is designed to maintain a constant temperature of around 98.6° Fahrenheit, regardless of surrounding environmental circumstances. The constancy of this temperature is necessary for the body to work efficiently. The body's mechanisms for regulating its temperature usually work very well under a wide variety of external conditions. Sometimes, however, the body is overwhelmed by extremes of cold too powerful for these mechanisms to counteract, and illness occurs.

It is possible for extremely low temperatures to occur in any location, indoors or outdoors. There are other factors, however, that can lead to or cause cold-related illness, even in the absence of extreme temperatures. These include humidity, wind, clothing, living and working conditions, physical activity, and an individual's health.

Cold-related illnesses are progressive and can, if unattended to, become life threatening. Once signs and symptoms appear, the victim's condition can deteriorate rapidly, leading to permanent injury or death.

When body temperature starts to drop, usually because of a drop in the temperature of the surrounding air, blood vessels near the skin contract and warm blood concentrates more toward the center of the body, so that less heat escapes through the skin. When this process is not sufficient to keep the body warm, shivering is triggered, which creates heat through muscle action.

Humidity increases the effects of cold by limiting the body's power to effectively maintain a stable temperature. A strong wind can also disastrously increase the effect of cold temperatures on the body. This combination of the cooling powers of low temperature and wind is called the *wind-chill factor.*

Obviously, sensitivity to extremes of cold can also be modulated by the kind of clothing you wear, how strenuous your physical activity is, how much and how often you drink liquids, and the duration of your exposure.

In addition, there are people who are particularly vulnerable to cold-related illness for a variety of reasons; these include:

- People who work or exercise strenuously outdoors
- The elderly and the very young
- Anyone with health problems
- People who have any condition that causes poor circulation, such as cardiovascular disease
- People who are taking diuretics (medications that eliminate water from the body)

What makes people particularly vulnerable is the inability to escape conditions of extreme cold, a failure to recognize the signs and symptoms, or an emotional involvement with an activity that leads them to ignore danger signals.

Frostbite and *hypothermia* are the two cold emergencies you will be most likely to encounter. Frostbite occurs to parts of the body that are over-exposed to cold, whereas hypothermia is a condition affecting the entire body when it can no longer generate enough heat to maintain normal temperature.

Frostbite, which is the freezing of body tissues, usually occurs in uncovered or lightly covered areas of the body in very low temperatures. It is more likely to occur when the wind is blowing, rapidly taking heat away from the body. Frostbite can be superficial, in which only the skin is frozen, or deep, in which the underlying tissues are also affected. As a result of exposure to cold, blood vessels constrict, so the blood supply to the chilled parts decreases and they do not get the warmth they need. The water in and between the body's cells freezes and swells, and the ice crystals and swelling damage or destroy the cells. Nose, cheeks, ears, toes, and fingers are the body parts most easily frostbitten. Fingers, hands, toes, feet, and legs can be lost as the result of tissue damage.

The signs and symptoms of frostbite, which goes through three stages of development, may not always be apparent to the victim. Since frostbite has a numbing effect, he might not be aware of it until told by someone.

Signs and Symptoms of Early Frostbite (Also Called Frostnip):

➤ The affected area feels numb to the victim; the numbness is possibly preceded by some pain.
➤ The skin becomes red, then white.

Treatment for Frostnip:

1. Place hand over frostnipped part.
2. Place frostnipped finger in armpit.

Signs and Symptoms of Superficial Frostbite:

➤ All pain disappears and the exposed surface becomes numb.
➤ Skin becomes white or grayish yellow and waxy.
➤ Skin feels very cold to the touch.
➤ Skin is firm to the touch, but the underlying tissues are soft.
➤ Blisters may form.

Treatment for Superficial Frostbite:

1. While outside, cover the frozen part with extra clothing or a warm cloth. If the hand or fingers are frostbitten, put the hand under the armpit for additional warmth.
2. *Do not rub the affected area with snow or anything else.* Rubbing causes further damage because of the sharp ice crystals in the skin.
3. Bring the victim inside promptly.
4. Rewarm the frostbitten area as rapidly as possible by gently soaking it in water the temperature

of which is 100° to 105° Fahrenheit. Test the water first with a thermometer, or if one is not available, with your forearm. If the water is uncomfortable to your touch, it is too warm. Do not let the affected part touch the bottom or sides of the container. Keep the injured area in the water until it feels warm, regains sensation, and appears red or pink, or, in the case of very dark skinned people, returns to its normal color and texture.

5. If water is not available, gently wrap the frostbitten part in blankets or other warm materials. Do *not* use heat lamps, hot water bottles, or heating pads. Do *not* allow the victim to place frostbitten areas near a hot stove or radiator. They can become burned before feeling returns.

6. Do *not* break any blisters.

7. Cover the area with a dry, sterile dressing. If the fingers or toes are frostbitten, place cotton or gauze between them.

8. Splint, if possible, if dealing with an extremity. Do *not* allow a victim with frostbitten toes to walk.

9. Elevate the frostbitten area.

10. Do *not* allow the victim to smoke or to drink coffee, tea, or hot chocolate, all activities that cause the blood vessels to constrict. Do *not* allow the victim to drink alcohol.

11. Seek medical attention promptly.

Signs and Symptoms of Deep Frostbite (Also Called Freezing):

➤ All sensation is lost.
➤ Skin becomes dead white or mottled blue-white. In

severe cases, the skin may be black, indicating that tissue has died. In very dark skinned victims, skin has a plastic, mottled look, clearly different from surrounding tissue.

➤ Skin and underlying tissues are firm to the touch.

Treatment for Deep Frostbite:

1. Cover the frostbitten area with a blanket or other warm materials.
2. Take the victim *without delay* to the nearest hospital emergency room.
3. If transport is delayed, rewarming may be done at the site as described above. Be aware that an extreme amount of pain may accompany rewarming. *Do not rewarm if there is any possibility of refreezing.*

Hypothermia is a general cooling of the entire body, to a point below 95° Fahrenheit. The inner core of the body is chilled and the body's warming mechanisms fail, so the body cannot generate heat to stay warm. As the body temperature cools, the heart starts to beat erratically (ventricular fibrillation) and eventually stops. If not given care, the victim will die.

Hypothermia can be produced by exposure to extremely low temperatures or to temperatures between 30° and 50° Fahrenheit with wind and rain. Fatigue, hunger, and poor physical condition can also contribute to the body's susceptibility to hypothermia. Thus, elderly people in poorly heated homes, particularly if they have poor nutrition and get little exercise, can develop hypothermia at higher temperatures. Certain substances, such as alcohol and barbiturates, can interfere with the body's normal response to cold, allowing hypothermia to occur more easily. Medical conditions such as infection, insulin reaction, stroke, and brain tumor also make a person more susceptible. Anyone remaining in cold water or in wet clothing for a long period of time may also be vulnerable. As the body starts losing heat faster than it can be produced, the resulting chilling takes the body through several stages:

1. Shivering. This is an involuntary adjustment by the body to preserve normal temperature in the vital organs by creating heat through muscular movement. This drains the body's energy reserves. Then the following stages occur:
2. Numbness
3. Apathy; listlessness; indifference; sleepiness; decreasing levels of judgment, reasoning powers, and consciousness; glassy, uncomprehending stare. These are the result of the cold reaching the brain
4. Slow, irregular pulse
5. Low body temperature
6. Weak or absent muscle coordination
7. Unconsciousness when the entire body is severely chilled or frozen

Be aware that the victim of hypothermia may not recognize its signs and symptoms and may deny that medical help is needed.

Treatment for Hypothermia:

1. Call EMS personnel.
2. Maintain an open airway and restore breathing if necessary (see p. 160).
3. Get the victim out of the elements, into a warm room, if possible.
4. Remove any wet clothing and dry the victim.
5. Wrap the victim in blankets or put on dry, warm clothing and move the victim to a warm environment. If using blankets, make certain that they go under as well as over the victim. Continue to warm the body gradually by building a fire or placing heat packs, electric heating pads, hot water bottles, or even another rescuer in the blankets with the victim. Always keep some barrier like a blanket, towel, or clothing between the heat source and the victim. Do *not* rewarm the victim too quickly, as by immersion in warm water. Rapid rewarming can be dangerous to heart rhythms. Handle the victim with extreme gentleness. In very severe cases, rough handling may result in death.
6. If the victim is conscious, give him or her warm (not hot) liquids to drink. Do *not* give the victim any alcoholic beverages.
7. If the victim is conscious, try to keep him or her awake.
8. Continue to monitor breathing and circulation. Be prepared to start cardiopulmonary resuscitation (CPR; see p. 229) if pulse stops.

Tips for Preventing Cold Injuries:

- Avoid being outdoors in the coldest part of the day.
- Avoid doing heavy exercise at the coldest part of the day.
- Alter your activity level according to the temperature, wind, and rain.
- Take frequent breaks to allow the body to readjust its temperature maintenance mechanisms.
- Dress appropriately for the environment and carry adequate waterproof clothing.
- Drink large amounts of fluids.
- Do *not* drink alcohol or take any drug or medication that might lower your awareness of temperature extremes if you are planning to be outdoors in extremely cold or wet weather.

Diabetic Emergencies

Body and brain cells need a wide variety of nutrients, of which one of the most critical is sugar. In digestion, the body breaks down various foods into sugar, which enters the bloodstream but cannot easily pass from the blood into cells without insulin, a chemical produced in the pancreas. When the balance between sugar and insulin is disturbed, the cells starve and the body cannot function normally. This condition is called *diabetes mellitus* or, more commonly, simply *diabetes*. There are between 11 million and 12 million diabetics in the United States.

There are two primary kinds of diabetes: type I, or insulin-dependant diabetes, and type II, or non-insulin-dependent diabetes. In type I, very little or no insulin is produced by the body and the diabetic must take daily injections of insulin, in addition to monitoring his or her diet and exercise. The condition tends to begin in childhood and is therefore often called juvenile diabetes. In type II, the body produces some insulin, but not enough for its needs. This can often be managed through careful monitoring of diet and exercise, and usually occurs in older adults. It is also called maturity-onset diabetes.

111

When a diabetic of either kind fails to control the insulin/sugar balance in his or her body, one of two problems can occur—too much or too little sugar in the bloodstream.

The condition in which the insulin level is too low and the sugar level too high is called *hyperglycemia*. In this condition, sugar is present in the blood but cannot get into the cells without insulin. The cells become starved for sugar, and the body attempts to meet its energy requirements by using other stored food and energy sources such as fats. Converting fat into energy produces waste products and increases the level of acidity in the blood, causing a condition called *acidosis*. The person becomes ill and, if the situation continues, goes into a diabetic coma. Hyperglycemia can occur when a diabetic does not take enough insulin, when a diabetic consumes more sugar than insulin can accommodate, when a person contracts an infection that affects insulin production, or when a person vomits or sustains fluid loss. The onset of these signs and symptoms of acute hyperglycemia tends to be gradual.

Signs and Symptoms of Acute Hyperglycemia (Diabetic Coma):

➤ Extreme thirst
➤ Warm, dry, sometimes reddened skin
➤ Deep, rapid, labored breathing
➤ Rapid, weak pulse
➤ Excessive urination
➤ Dry mouth and tongue
➤ Drowsiness

➤ Nausea and vomiting with upper abdominal discomfort or pain
➤ Sickly sweet odor of acetone (similar to nail polish remover or spoiled fruit) on the breath
➤ A state of confusion and disorientation similar to drunkenness
➤ A coma state

Treatment for Diabetic Coma:

1. If the victim is unconscious, maintain an open airway (see p. 160) and call EMS personnel immediately.
2. If the victim is conscious, watch for vomiting and maintain an open airway. Ask the victim if he or she is diabetic or look for a Medic Alert tag. Then call EMS personnel.
3. Treat for shock (see p. 305).

Hypoglycemia is a condition in which the insulin level in the body is too high and the sugar level too low, leading in the diabetic to an extreme situation known as insulin shock. This can happen when the victim has not eaten adequately, so that not enough sugar has been taken in; the victim has taken too much insulin; the victim has overexercised, thus burning sugar too fast to be replaced; or the victim is suddenly put under great emotional stress. Note that the onset of hypoglycemia tends to be quite sudden.

Signs and Symptoms of Extreme Hypoglycemia (Insulin Shock):

➤ In the early stages, the victim may seem to experience a personality change, becoming excited, confused, and/or belligerent.

- Headache
- Profuse perspiration
- Hunger, but no thirst
- Cold, clammy, pale skin
- Dizziness
- Breathing normal or shallow
- Rapid, weak pulse
- Eventually, convulsions and unconsciousness

Even people who are accustomed to living with diabetics can encounter emergency situations that seem overwhelming, as 6-year-old Samantha Barth of Federal Way, Washington, discovered one afternoon in June 1992.

Samantha had been looking forward all day to spending the afternoon with her father, Nels. But as he was driving her home from the day-care center, she began to worry that something was serious wrong. "My daddy picked me up from the day-care," Samantha said, "and he was driving real fast and he was going in lanes that he wasn't supposed to be in. When we got home, he was just sitting in the car. I had to get out and pull him out." She tugged at her father's hand until he sluggishly stepped out of the car.

"You all right?" Samantha asked.

"Yeah," her father responded listlessly.

"I didn't know what was happening to Daddy, and he was acting real weird," Samantha said. Samantha's father went to lie down on the couch, while she turned on the television set and began watching it from a chair nearby.

"Are you okay, Daddy?" she asked anxiously, after a few minutes.

"Yeah," her father mumbled.

"Daddy, I think it's time for something to eat," Samantha said.

"Sometimes my daddy has problems with his blood sugar," she later explained, "so I thought I should get him something to eat. I climbed up on a chair to get the oranges and the chips. I thought about honey, but I said, 'No, it's too much of a mess.' I tried giving him an orange, but he wouldn't eat it. He said he didn't like oranges, but he does."

Samantha touched her father's forearm and felt the cold wetness of his skin. "Dad, you're sweaty," she said.

"My mom told me that you've always got to check his wrist to see if he's sweaty or not," Samantha explained. "If he's sweaty, he's either low or high. And so I just had to save his life." Samantha immediately dialed 9-1-1.

"Fire Department, Medic One, what is the address of the problem?" asked Federal Way fire dispatcher Pat Everett, who took the call.

"I have to go outside and look. Is that okay?" asked Samantha.

"Yes," said Everett.

Samantha came back to the phone with the address.

"Is that where you're calling?"

"Yes."

"And that's where the problem is?"

"Yes."

"Okay, what's the matter?"

"I think my daddy is low," Samantha said, "and he's a diabetic."

"You think he's low?" Everett asked, to be certain she was getting the information correctly.

"When she told me that her daddy was low and that he was a diabetic, the first thing I was thinking was that I hope he's not truly unconscious and that this man needs CPR," Everett said.

"Is he awake?" she asked Samantha.

"No."

"He's not awake?"

"No."

"How old are you?"

"I'm 6½," Samantha answered.

"You're 6½ and you're there by yourself?"

"Yes."

"Okay, can you go over there and shake your daddy and see if he'll wake up?" Everett asked.

"Okay."

"Okay, you go over there and shake him. I have help on the way, but don't hang up. Go shake him and see if he wakes up, okay?"

"Okay."

"And come back to the phone," Everett said.

"If he wakes up, do you want to talk to him then?" Samantha asked.

"You just see if you can wake him up—shake him hard," Everett said. "You go do that and then come back to the phone."

Rescue units were immediately dispatched, including King County paramedic Chris Merritt. "Insulin shock can rapidly progress to complete coma," Merritt said, "and if sugar is not administered orally or intravenously, the patient will die."

"It's scary being all alone with your daddy and nobody with you, when he's low on sugar," Samantha said. She went back to her father and began shaking him and calling out "Daddy! Daddy!" as loudly as she could. Although he grunted in response, he did not awaken. She went back to the phone to report her failure.

Everett relayed the information to the rescuers en route, as another dispatcher took over talking to Samantha. "Listen carefully now," he told her. "The aid car is on its way over there already."

"I just can't wait till my mom gets home," Samantha said. "I'm real scared."

"They'll be right there to see you, okay?"

"Okay."

"You did a good job, honey," the dispatcher told her.

"Now can I call my mom?" Samantha asked.

"Yes," he said.

Within 3 minutes of the call, the first rescue units arrived on the scene. "When the medics came, I was hoping they would make him feel better," Samantha said.

Lieutenant Robert Shinnett, an EMT, took charge. "When we arrived at the scene, it was just at the point where he was going to start to be more critical," Stinnett said. "Nels, we're going to put some glucose in your mouth. Can you hear me all right?" he asked Samantha's father, who grunted to indicate that he had heard what was said to him. "He was able to take a little bit of it orally, but obviously he was so far out that he needed more medical attention," Shinnett said he concluded. Moments later, the advanced life-support unit arrived. "We knew what the problem was, but we needed to confirm it," Shinnett said. "We found his blood sugar to be at 20, which is extremely low—dangerously low, in fact. A normal blood sugar is about 120. So we administered two intravenous doses of $D_{50}W$, which is a highly concentrated sugar solution, and within just minutes, he was alert and oriented and thanking us for waking him up." Samantha began bring her father things to eat to bring his blood sugar up even farther.

"The problem I had that day definitely threw me," Nels later said. "I knew there was something wrong, but I had mistaken having low blood sugar for just being fatigued. Samantha just did a fantastic job."

"If her parents had not educated her on the signs and symptoms of insulin shock, I'm sure he would have lain there and died," Stinnett said.

"Samantha was just fabulous," said her mother. "She saw that Daddy was in an obvious diabetic state, that he was having a crisis. She assessed the situation and took immediate action. She's 6½ years old—she's one in a million."

"They fixed him all up and then it was all over with, and then I lay down on the couch and went to sleep and then Mommy came home," Samantha said.

The fire department later presented Samantha with an award for saving her father's life. "To think that a 6-year-old can pick up a phone and dial 9-1-1 and be able to explain the symptoms of a disease is amazing. I'm very proud of Samantha," her mother said.

"I'm surprised that Samantha reacted the way that she did, and obviously relieved," said her father. "I think pride in my daughter is almost an understatement there."

"Just because they're children does not mean that they cannot react in the face of an emergency," said dispatcher Everett. "They're a lot more receptive than we think they are. We don't give them enough credit."

"I'm happier than anything in the whole entire world," said Samantha, "because I saved my daddy's life and I love him infinity."

Treatment for Extreme Hypoglycemia
(Insulin Shock):

1. If the victim is conscious, give sugar in the form of candy, fruit juice, nondiet soft drinks, straight table sugar, or table sugar dissolved in water or juice. Don't worry about giving too much sugar, since medical professionals will balance it with the proper amount of insulin if necessary when they arrive. *Note:* If you cannot distinguish between a victim with insulin shock and a victim progressing into a diabetic coma, give sugar to the victim. Giving sugar to a victim with too much blood sugar will not make a significant difference in the outcome, whereas giving sugar to a victim of insulin shock could save his or her life.
2. If the victim is unconscious, a "sprinkle" of granulated sugar can be placed under the tongue. Monitor breathing and maintain body temperature.
3. If the victim is unconscious, or is conscious but does not feel better within 5 minutes of consuming sugar, call EMS personnel immediately.
4. All victims of insulin shock should be seen by a physician.

Dislocations and Fractures

Dislocations

A dislocation occurs when one or more of the bones forming a joint slips out of its normal position. This most often happens to the so-called freely moveable joints of the lower jaw, the shoulders, the elbows, the wrists, the fingers, the hips, the knees, the ankles, and the toes. Dislocations are caused by some force pushing the ends of the bones far enough beyond their normal range of motion to stretch or tear the ligaments holding them in place. This may be the result of a force applied at or near the point, a sudden muscular contraction, a twisting strain on the ligaments, or a fall in which the force of the landing is transferred to a joint (as when one attempts to "break" a fall by putting out a hand, which can cause dislocation in the finger or wrist). The violence of a dislocating force may also cause a fracture and damage nerves and blood vessels in the area.

A dislocation is probably the easiest musculo-skeletal injury to identify because of the deformity of the joint caused by the displacement of the bone end from its normal position.

121

General Signs and Symptoms of Dislocations:

➤ Abnormal bump, ridge, or depression at the joint
➤ Rigidity and loss of function
➤ Pain upon attempting to move the joint
➤ Tenderness to the touch
➤ Swelling
➤ Discoloration

Physicians generally advise against trying to put a dislocated bone back into place unless you are professionally trained to do this, because of the danger of further damaging ligaments, blood vessels, and nerves found close to the joints. The general rule is to immobilize the injured joint by splinting it in the line of deformity in which you find it, and to obtain medical help. A splint is a device used to immobilize a body part, and there are a variety of splints available commercially. They can also be improvised from pieces of wood, broom handles, newspapers, heavy cardboard, boards, magazines, or similar firm materials. See the guidelines for splinting in the section on fractures that begins on p. 127.

Dislocation of a Shoulder

Shoulder dislocations usually occur as the result of falls or blows directly on the shoulder or by falls on the hands and elbows. They can take 3 to 6 weeks to heal.

Signs and Symptoms of a Shoulder Dislocation:

➤ The elbow stands 1 or 2 inches away from the body, and the victim cannot bring it in contact with his side.
➤ The arm is held rigid.
➤ The shoulder appears flat.
➤ A marked depression can be seen beneath the point of the shoulder.
➤ The shoulder is painful and swollen.

Treatment for a Dislocated Shoulder:

Supporting the arm in the position in which it was found, immobilize it in the following manner:

1. Place the point of a wedge-shaped pad, approximately 4 inches wide and 1 to 3 inches thick, between the injured arm and the body, above the elbow, and tape or tie it in place.
2. Apply an ice pack or cold compress to reduce the swelling and inhibit internal bleeding.
3. Seek medical help.

Dislocation of the Elbow

The most common causes of an elbow dislocation are a blow to the elbow or, more rarely, a fall on the hand. Since all the nerves and blood vessels that go to the forearm and the hand pass through the elbow, any injury to this joint can be extremely serious and, if not treated properly, can cause permanent disability.

Signs and Symptoms of a Dislocated Elbow:

➤ Deformity at the elbow
➤ Inability to bend the arm at the elbow
➤ Intense pain

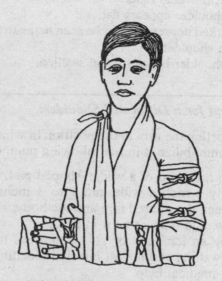

Splint for Dislocation of Wrist

Dislocation of the Wrist

A dislocation of the wrist usually occurs when a hand is extended to break a fall. It is usually difficult to distinguish between a wrist dislocation and fractured wrist, so a suspected dislocation should be treated as if it were a fracture (see p. 139).

Dislocation of the Finger or Toe

Signs and Symptoms of a Dislocated Finger or Toe:

➤ Inability to bend the dislocated joint
➤ Deformity of the joint
➤ Pain and swelling at the joint
➤ Shortening of the finger or toe

Immobilize the digit by using small pads to cushion the deformity and splinting, or by tying it to an adjoining digit. An ice-cream stick makes an excellent finger splint.

Dislocation of the Hip

Dislocation of the hip usually occurs from falling onto the foot or knee. It can also be the result of a direct blow to the hip, when the thigh is extended at an angle to the spine.

Signs and Symptoms of a Dislocated Hip:

➤ Intense pain
➤ Lengthening or shortening of the leg, with the foot turned in or out
➤ Pain and swelling at the joint

Dislocation of the Knee

Dislocations of the knee occur from direct force applied at the knee or from a fall on the knee. Knee injuries are common in sports that involve quick movements or exert unusual force on the knee.

Signs and Symptoms of Knee Dislocation:

➤ Deformity
➤ Inability to use the knee
➤ Intense pain

Supporting the dislocation, apply a splint as for a fracture of the thigh (see pp. 146–47), using either a broken-back splint or a stretcher board. Place extra padding of blankets, clothes, or similar materials to conform to the deformity.

If the knee is bent and cannot be straightened, support it in the bent position by having the victim rest it on a pillow.

Dislocation of the Ankle

Various types of deformity may be symptomatic of an ankle dislocation, and when the ankle is dislocated, bones are almost always broken. There is usually rapid and very noticeable swelling and intense pain.

Supporting the dislocation, apply an improvised splint as for a fracture of the ankle or foot (see pp. 149–50), adding padding to conform to the deformity. Use an air splint long enough to immobilize the knee or use a blanket or pillow to splint the leg or ankle. Use additional cravats for anchoring to a broken-back splint.

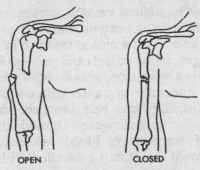

OPEN   CLOSED

Open and Closed Fractures

Fractures

A fracture is a break, a crack, or a crushing of the bone. There are two kinds of fractures: (1) open, or compound, and (2) closed, or simple. In an open fracture, the bone is broken and an open wound is created, extending down to the bone, sometimes with the bone sticking out through the wound. This often occurs when a limb is severely bent, so that the broken ends of the bone tear the skin and surrounding soft tissue. It also occurs when an object penetrates the skin, breaking the bone. In a closed fracture, the bone is broken or cracked, but there is no open wound. Open fractures are usually more dangerous because of the possibility of heavy bleeding and the threat of infection.

Although fractures are rarely immediately life threatening, a fracture to a large bone can cause the victim to go into severe shock because the bone itself and surrounding soft tissue may bleed heavily. Broken bones, particularly the long bones of the arms and legs, often have sharp, saw-toothed edges that can cut into blood vessels, nerves, or muscles with the slightest movement. Careless or improper handling can convert a closed fracture into an open one, damaging blood vessels and nerves in the process, creating a much more serious injury and leaving the victim vulnerable to greater pain and shock. The period of disability may be prolonged, and the victim's life may be endangered through the hemorrhaging of surrounding blood vessels. Fracture victims should therefore be handled with extreme caution.

Signs and Symptoms of a Fracture:

➤ Pain or tenderness in the region of the fracture, particularly when touched or moved

➤ Deformity of the affected area—check to see if it is different in shape or length from the same bone on the opposite side of the body.

➤ Moderate or severe swelling

➤ Bluish discoloration

➤ Injured part moves unnaturally or abnormally.

➤ Victim reports having heard bone snap or crack.

➤ Victim feels grating sensation of bone ends rubbing together.

➤ Victim or bystander reports a manner in which injury occurred that is suggestive of a fracture.

Determine whether to call EMS personnel or to transport the person to a doctor's office or emergency department in a hospital. Call EMS immediately if this is deemed necessary. No attempt should be made to change the position of the injured person until you have determined that movement will not complicate the injury. If the victim is lying down, it is best to attend to his or her injuries while he or she is in that position. Maintain an open airway (see p. 160), control bleeding (see p. 37). As with strains and sprains, *rest, ice,* and *elevation* are the general rule. If movement is absolutely necessary, protect the injured part against further injury, usually by splinting. In general, however, it is best not to move the victim. Do *not* attempt to push any part of an exposed bone back into the wound. Do not wash the wound or insert anything, including medication, into it.

Splints are used to immobilize and protect areas with musculoskeletal injuries such as known or suspected fractures, dislocations, or severe sprains. *When in doubt, treat the injury as a fracture and splint it.* Splints prevent movement at the area of the injury and the nearest joint. They should immobilize the joint or bones above and below the break. They ease pain, keep the break from becoming worse, and help prevent shock. The most common types of commercially available splints are air (inflatable) splints, board splints, and flexible splints. You are more likely to use splints made from materials readily available around the home. There are splints that use soft materials, splints that use rigid materials, and the body itself, used as a splint. Soft splints can be made made from folded blankets, pillows, towels, wadded sheets, or other cloth. A sling is a kind of soft splint made from a triangular or cravat bandage (see p. 51) used to support an arm, wrist, or hand. Rigid splints can be made from boards, folded magazines, strips of metal, and similar materials. The body can also be used as a splint

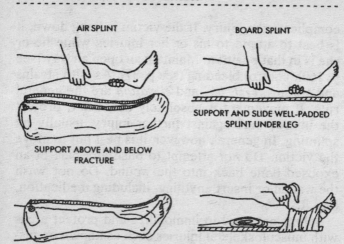

AIR SPLINT

SUPPORT ABOVE AND BELOW
FRACTURE

BOARD SPLINT

SUPPORT AND SLIDE WELL-PADDED
SPLINT UNDER LEG

APPLY SPLINT TO LIMB
AND INFLATE

PAD SPACES BETWEEN LEG AND SPLINT
AND BANDAGE SECURELY

Splinting

by binding an injured part to an uninjured part, such
as an injured arm to the chest, or an injured leg to
an uninjured leg.

Use the following guidelines when splinting a suspected fracture or dislocation:

1. Splint only if you can do so without causing
   more pain and discomfort to the victim.
2. Gently remove all clothing from any suspected
   fracture or dislocation.
3. Do *not* attempt to straighten any fracture or to
   push bones back through an open wound.
4. Cover any open wounds with a sterile dressing
   before splinting.
5. Splint an injury in the direction in which you
   find it.

6. Pad splints with soft material to prevent excessive pressure on the affected area and to aid in supporting the injured part.

7. Pad under the natural arches of the body such as the knee and wrist.

8. Support the injured part while the splint is being applied.

9. Splint the injured area and the joints above and below the injured site.

10. Splint firmly but not so tightly as to interfere with circulation or cause undue pain.

11. Check circulation before and after splinting by looking at fingers or toes and by questioning the victim. Loosen the splint if the victim complains of numbness or if fingers or toes turn blue or become cold.

12. Support or immobilize the fracture before transporting the victim.

13. Elevate the injured part if possible.

14. Apply ice or a cold pack.

Fracture of the Collarbone

The collarbone or clavicle is the most frequently injured bone in the shoulder, and is more often fractured in children than adults. The most frequent cause of a collarbone fracture is a fall on an outstretched hand, although it can also be caused by a blow to the shoulder.

Signs and Symptoms of a Broken Collarbone:

➤ Pain in the shoulder area, sometimes radiating down the arm

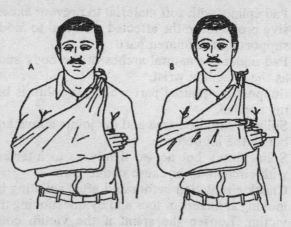

Bandage for a Fracture of the Collarbone

➤ Partial or total disability of the arm on the injured side
➤ Injured shoulder droops forward
➤ Victim frequently supports the arm on the injured side at the elbow or wrist with the other hand, holding it against the chest

Because the collarbone lies over major blood vessels and the nerves to the arm, it is important to immobilize it to prevent damage to these tissues. Support the fracture until the following dressings have been applied:

1. Place padding between the arm on the injured side and the victim's side.
2. Secure the arm to the body with a medium cravat (see p. 311). Center the bandage on the outside

of the arm. Carry the ends of the bandage across the chest and back and tie over a pad on the uninjured side of the body.

3. Alternatively, use an elastic bandage or strip of cloth to make a figure-eight bandage around the victim's shoulders, back, and chest.

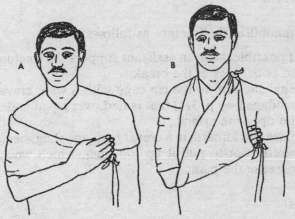

Bandage for Fracture of the Upper Third of the Arm

Fracture of the Upper Arm

The humerus, the bone of the upper arm, is the largest bone in the arm. Fractures of the humerus usually occur at the upper end, near the shoulder, or in the middle of the bone. Upper-end fractures are more common in the elderly and young children, usually as the result of a fall. Fractures in the middle of the humerus more often occur in young adults.

Signs and Symptoms of a Fracture in the Middle of the Humerus:

➤ Swelling
➤ Deformity
➤ Inability to use the arm below the point of the fracture

Immobilize the fracture as follows:

1. If possible, have an assistant support the fracture on both sides of the break.
2. Bind the arm to the rib cage with a wide cravat bandage (see p. 311) that is tied over a pad under the opposite armpit.
3. Place the forearm in a cravat bandage sling, being careful not to pull it up too high, which would increase the pain.

Or:

1. Place some light padding in the victim's armpit.
2. Gently place the arm at the victim's side, with the forearm at a right angle across the victim's chest.
3. Make a padded splint out of newspaper or other material.
4. Support the forearm at the wrist with a narrow sling tied around the neck.
5. Bind the upper arm to the victim's body by placing a large towel, bed sheet, or other cloth around

the splint and the victim's chest and tying it under the opposite arm.
6. Keep the victim sitting up while transporting him or her to a medical facility.

Fracture of the Elbow

As with dislocations of the elbow, fractures must be dealt with very carefully because of the possibility of extensive damage to surrounding tissues, nerves, and blood vessels. Improper care and handling could result in permanent disability.

Signs and Symptoms of a Fractured Elbow:

➤ Extreme pain
➤ Extensive discoloration around the elbow
➤ Deformity
➤ Bone may be visible or projecting from the wound

If the victim says that he or she cannot move the elbow, do not attempt to move it. Immobilize it in the position in which you find it and call EMS personnel immediately. Immobilize a fracture elbow when the arm is found in a *straight* position as follows:

1. Do not bend, straighten, or twist the arm in any direction.
2. If available, apply an inflatable plastic splint.
3. If an inflatable splint is not available, use a splint long enough to reach from 1 inch below the armpit to 1 inch beyond the tip of the middle finger.
4. While the fracture is being supported, pad it to conform to the deformity and place the splint on the inner side of the arm.

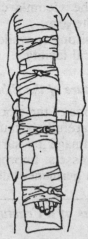

**Bandage for Fracture of Elbow
in Straight Position**

5. Prepare five cravat bandages (see pp. 51 and 311).
6. Place the center of the first cravat bandage on the outside of the arm at the upper end of the splint, cross over the splint on the inside of the arm, pass the ends one or more times around the arm and the splint and tie on the outside of the arm.
7. Place the center of the second cravat bandage on the outside of the arm just above the elbow and tie the same way.
8. Repeat the process with the third cravat bandage on the forearm, just below the elbow.
9. Place the center of the fourth cravat bandage on the back of the wrist, passing the ends around the splint and under the wrist. Bring one end up around the little finger side and cross it

over the back of the hand and down between the forefinger and the thumb. Bring the other end around over the thumb, across the back of the hand, and over the little finger side. Cross both ends under the wrist and tie them together at the back of the hand.

10. Bind the limb to the body with the fifth cravat bandage.

If the arm is *bent*, immobilize it in the bent position by making an L-shaped splint for the forearm and wrist from two pieces of board ¼ inch thick and 4 inches wide. One piece should be long enough to extend from 1 inch below the armpit to the point of the elbow and the other long enough to extend from the point of the elbow to 1 inch beyond the end of the middle finger. Immobilize the arm to the splint as in the following manner:

1. Fasten the boards together securely to form an L-shaped splint.
2. Pad the splint.
3. While an assistant supports the fracture on both sides of the break, place the forearm across the chest and apply the splint to the inner side of the arm and forearm.
4. Prepare four cravat bandages (see pp. 51 and 311) to hold the splint in place.
5. Place the center of the first cravat bandage on the outside of the arm at the upper end of the splint, pass around the arm one or more times, and tie on the arm.
6. Place the centers of the second and third cravat bandages on the upper arm and the forearm—

above and below the elbow, respectively—pass around one or more times, and tie on the arm.

7. Place the center of a fourth cravat bandage on the back of the wrist, passing the ends around the splint and under the wrist. Bring one end up around the little finger side and cross it over the back of the hand and down between the forefinger and the thumb. Bring the other end around over the thumb, across the back of the hand, and over the little finger side. Cross both ends under the wrist and tie them together at the back of the hand.

8. Place the arm in a cravat bandage sling.

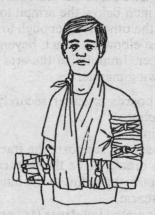

Splint for Lower Two-thirds of Arm, Elbow, Forearm, or Wrist

Fractures of the Forearm and Wrist

Fractures of the forearm and wrist are usually less painful than those of the upper arm, shoulder blade, or elbow. The two forearm bones, the radius and the ulna, are more commonly fractured in children than in adults, usually from falling on an outstretched arm. Because these bones are near the radial artery and nerve, their fracture may cause severe bleeding or the inability to move the wrist and hand.

Signs and Symptoms of a Forearm and Wrist Fracture:

➤ Pain
➤ Tenderness to the touch
➤ Severe deformity, especially if both forearm bones are broken, giving the forearm a characteristic S shape

If available, use a plastic inflatable splint to immobilize the forearm or wrist. If not:

1. Carefully place the lower arm at a right angle across the victim's chest, with the palm facing toward the chest and the thumb pointing upward.
2. Support the injured part by placing a splint underneath the forearm, extending it beyond both the hand and the elbow. Padded newspapers or magazines wrapped around the arm on both sides can also be used.
3. Place a roll of gauze or similar object in the palm to keep the hand and fingers in a normal position.
4. Secure the splint with cravats or roller gauze above and below the break.
5. Put the arm in a sling with the hand 3 to 4 inches above the level of the elbow and secure it to the chest with cravats.

6. Elevate and apply an ice pack or cold compress.
7. Transport the victim to a medical facility in a sitting position for comfort.

Fracture of the Hand

Fractures of the hand are usually caused by a direct blow.

Signs and Symptoms of a Hand Fracture:

➤ Acute pain
➤ Tenderness to the touch
➤ Swelling
➤ Discoloration
➤ Enlarged joints

If available, a plastic inflatable splint can be used to immobilize the injury. If not, use a board splint and proceed as follows:

1. Place a well-padded splint—about ¼ inch thick, 4 inches wide, and long enough to reach from the point of the elbow to 1 inch beyond the middle finger—under the forearm.
2. Place padding, like a roll of gauze or similar object, in the palm to keep the palm and the fingers in a normal position, and additional padding under the wrist.
3. Apply the splint to the inside of the forearm and hand with one cravat and one triangular bandage as described in steps 4 through 8 (see pp. 50–51).
4. Place the center of the cravat on the outside of the arm just below the elbow. Pass it around

the forearm one or more times and tie it on the outside of the forearm.

5. Place the base of a triangular bandage (the longest side) under the splint at the wrist. Bring the apex (the point opposite the base, where the two other sides meet) around the end of the splint over the hand to a point above the wrist.

6. Carry one end around the little finger side across the back of the hand and wrist and the other end around the thumb side across the back of the hand and wrist.

7. Cross the end on the inside of the wrist, bring them to the back of the wrist, and tie.

8. Bring the apex down over the knot and tuck it under. Alternatively, the splint may be fastened to the arm with two cravat bandages or two roller bandages.

9. Place the forearm in a cravat bandage sling.

10. Bind the arm to the chest with cravats.

11. Apply ice and take the victim to a hospital.

Fracture of the Fingers

Signs and Symptoms of a Finger Fracture:

➤ Pain
➤ Swelling
➤ Deformity

To immobilize:

1. Place a narrow padded splint, like an ice-cream stick, under the finger and the palm of the hand.

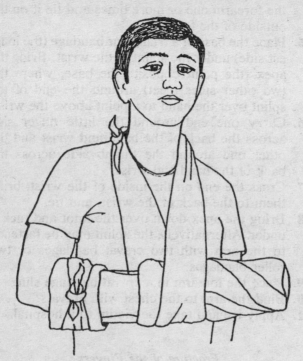

**Dressing for Fracture or Crushed Bones of
the Hand or Fingers**

2. Fasten the splint to the hand with three strips of
   cloth, tied over the splint, or with three pieces
   of tape, one crossing the hand and the palm, one
   on the finger above the fracture, and one on the
   finger below the fracture.
3. Place the hand in a sling.
4. Elevate and apply ice.

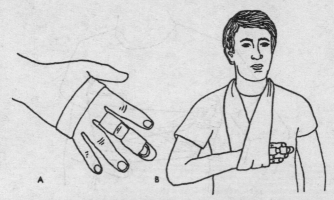

Bandage for Fracture of a Finger

Rib Fractures

Rib fractures are generally caused by a direct blow or severe squeezing. The rib can fracture at any point along the bone. Although painful, a simple rib fracture is rarely life threatening.

Signs and Symptoms of a Rib Fracture:

➤ Severe pain on breathing, which worsens with deep breathing
➤ Shallow breathing to avoid pain
➤ Instinctive support of the injured area with the victim's hand or arm to ease the pain
➤ Tenderness over the fracture
➤ Deformity

Treatment for a Fractured Rib:

1. Put the victim in a position that will make breathing easier.

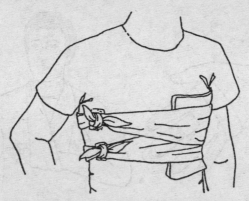

Bandage for Fracture of a Rib

2. Bind the victim's arm to the chest on the injured side, or use a pillow or rolled blanket to support and immobilize the area, or:

   a. Apply padding over the injured ribs, and bind to the chest with two medium cravat bandages, centered just above and below the pain.
   b. When the victim exhales, tie the bandages with knots on the opposite side of the chest.
   c. Support the arm on the injured side with a sling.

3. Apply ice.
4. Monitor breathing and pulse.
5. Treat for shock (see p. 305).
6. Call EMS personnel or transport the victim to a medical facility.

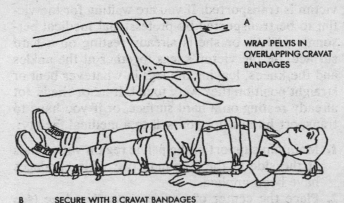

WRAP PELVIS IN
OVERLAPPING CRAVAT
BANDAGES

B   SECURE WITH 8 CRAVAT BANDAGES

Immobilized Fractured Pelvis or Hip

Fracture of the Pelvis or Hip

A fracture of the pelvis or the hip usually results from a squeezing or crushing type injury or from a direct blow. There may be associated injuries to the digestive, urinary, or genital organs, so extreme care should be used in handling the victim.

Signs and Symptoms of a Pelvic or Hip Fracture:

➤ Pain in the pelvic region
➤ Discoloration
➤ Inability to raise the leg
➤ Inward rotation of foot and leg on the affected side

Keep the victim lying down on his or her back. The pelvic region should be supported before the victim is transported. If you are waiting for the victim to be transported by professional medical personnel and he or she is already resting on a hard surface, tie the victim's legs together at the ankles and the knees, leaving the legs in whatever bent or straight position they were found. If he or she is not already resting on a hard surface, or if you have to transport him or her yourself to a medical facility:

1. Maintain support of the pelvic region with hands at the side of the hips until two wide bandages have been applied.
2. Place the center of a wide cravat bandage (see pp. 51 and 311) over one hip, with the upper end extending about 2 inches above the hipbone.
3. Pass the bandage ends around the body and tie over a pad on the opposite hip.
4. Place the center of another wide cravat bandage on the other hip, and secure in the same fashion, tying it over the first bandage.
5. Lift the victim only high enough to place on a firm support, preferably a broken-back splint.
6. Treat for shock (see p. 305).

Fracture of the Thigh

The thighbone, or femur, is large and strong because (along with the bones of the lower leg) it must bear the body's weight, and for this reason a great deal of force is required to fracture it. A fracture of the femur can injure the femoral artery, which is the major supplier of blood to the leg, and the blood loss can be life threatening. Fractures of the thigh-

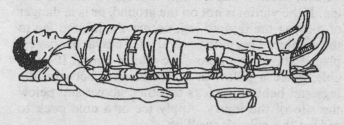

Splint for Fracture of the Thigh or Knee

bone usually occur at the upper end, where it meets the pelvis.

When the fracture occurs, the thigh muscles contract. They are so strong that they pull the broken bone ends together, causing them to overlap. This may cause the injured leg to shorten noticeably, and it may be turned outward.

Signs and Symptoms of a Broken Femur:

➤ Deformity, with the injured leg shorter than the other and turned out
➤ Severe pain
➤ Inability to move the leg

Since the person cannot walk to a car, it is best to call EMS personnel immediately, and then to immobilize the injury in the direction of the deformity and help the person to rest in a comfortable position. The ground is an excellent splint for any kind of leg injury, and a person found injured on the ground should not be moved. If there is an open wound, dress it and control bleeding before splinting. If the victim is not on the ground, or is in danger of moving the injured leg, secure the injured leg to the uninjured leg with several wide cravat bandages, placed above and below the site of injury. If available, place a pillow or rolled blanket between the legs and behind the legs together, above and below the site of the injury. Apply ice or a cold pack to reduce the pain or swelling.

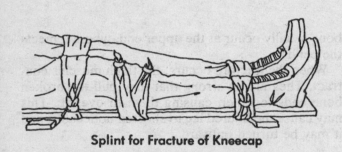

Splint for Fracture of Kneecap

Fractures of the Knee

The bones that form the joint of the knee—the lower end of the femur, the upper ends of the tibia and fibula, and the patella, or kneecap—are very vulnerable to injury. The kneecap, which lies directly beneath the skin and moves freely on the lower surface of the thighbone, can be broken by a violent force to the front of the knee or by falling and landing on bent knees. If the victim is on the ground, the knee is bent, and the victim cannot straighten it without pain, you can support a fracture of the kneecap or another part of the knee joint by putting a pillow under the knee and using the ground as a splint. If the knee is straight or can be straightened without pain, secure it to the uninjured leg as you would do for a fracture of the thigh and apply ice or a cold compress. Help the victim rest in as comfortable a position as possible, and call EMS personnel to have him or her transported to a medical facility.

Fractures of the Lower Leg

Treat fractures of the lower leg as you would fractures of the thigh.

Fractures of the Ankle or Foot

Fractures of the ankle or foot, like other injuries to these areas, can be caused by twisting forces. They can also occur from forcefully landing on the heel, as in a fall from a great height.

If pain, swelling, or inaccessible bleeding make it necessary to remove a boot or shoe, do so very carefully by unlacing or cutting the footwear in order to prevent further damage to the area. If there is no severe pain, swelling, or bleeding, it may be better to leave the boot or shoe on for additional support. You can improvise a splint for the ankle or foot as follows:

1. Keep the victim lying down, on his or her back.
2. Place a pillow or a folded blanket under the foot and the ankle and fold it around so the edges meet at the front of the leg.
3. Fasten the pillow or the blanket to the leg with

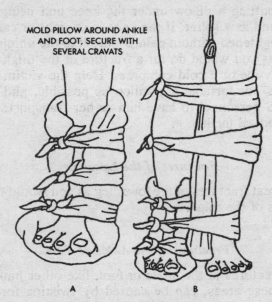

MOLD PILLOW AROUND ANKLE
AND FOOT, SECURE WITH
SEVERAL CRAVATS

A   B

Immobilized Ankle or Foot

three bandages: one above the ankle, one around
the ankle, and one below the ankle.
4. Fold the end of the padding that extends beyond
   the heel so that it supports the foot.
5. Apply ice.
6. Call EMS personnel and keep the victim from
   moving until they arrive.

Many sprains, strains, dislocations, and fractures
occur as the result of falls in the home, and nearly
half of all accidents in the home are due to falls.
The percentage is even higher among the elderly.

Tips for Preventing Dislocations and Fractures

- Make sure you do not have frayed carpets or loose banisters.
- Put nonskid underpads on all scatter rugs and area rugs or secure them with double-sided tape.
- Put nonskid strips in bathtubs that are used for showering and in shower stalls.
- Do not leave toys or other objects near the stairs.
- Do not carry large objects up or down stairs in such a way that you cannot see the steps beneath your feet.
- Put nonslip treads on indoor and outdoor wooden steps, or use paint mixed with sand for the final coating on outdoor steps.
- Use safety straps on highchairs and strollers to prevent babies from climbing out and falling.
- If you have children, make sure that the posts supporting the banisters of any staircases are too close together for them to fall through.
- Do not place furniture in front of a window that can be opened. Children may climb onto the furniture and fall through or out the window.
- Place window guards on upper-story windows to which children have access.
- Keep the outside of your house well lit at night. This will both prevent falls and discourage intruders.
- Use a night light so you won't trip in the dark.
- Keep your stairs well lit, with a light switch at the top and bottom of the staircase.

- Never leave a baby unattended on a bed, table, or other elevated surface.
- Clean up spills promptly.
- Make sure your balcony is childproof. Falls from second stories are a leading cause of injury among children under 5 years of age.

Drowning
(With General Instructions for Breathing Emergencies)

Drowning is a kind of suffocation in which the supply of air to the lungs has been cut off completely by water or spasm of the larynx due to submersion in water. Drowning starts when small amounts of water are drawn into the lungs by a person whose nose and throat are submerged. This causes the muscles of the larynx (voice box) to spasm, which closes the airway to keep more water from entering the lungs. Since these spasms also prevent air from entering, the victim suffocates and becomes unconscious. In unconsciousness the muscles relax, and the victim automatically breathes and draws more water into the lungs.

The cutoff of air does not immediately create a lack of oxygen in the body. There are small reserves in the air cells of the lungs, the blood, and some of the tissue, which can sustain life for up to 6 minutes or more in low temperatures (under 70° Fahrenheit). A reflex, strongest in young children, slows the heart rate and reserves oxygen in the blood for the heart and brain. This often permits people who have been submerged to survive without brain damage. Because this oxygen supply is used up so rapidly, however, it is essential to start artificial ventilation (rescue breathing) as soon as possible.

Every year, more than 2,000 young children in the United States die in drowning incidents. Dana Treganowan and Paula Haskell are two people who discovered to their horror just how easily a child who is not carefully watched can become a drowning victim.

Dana Treganowan never had any trouble getting her two young daughters—Laura, 2, and Caroline, 11 months—to take a bath. "When they were cranky, that was always something good to do with them, because they liked playing in the water," she said. "In fact, it was always a struggle to get them out of the tub."

On one evening in June 1991, after her husband left the house to do some construction work while it was still light out, Dana decided to bathe the girls, putting Caroline in the floater ring she had used with her since she was 6 months old and could sit up, while Laura played in the water at the shallow end of the tub. "I usually don't leave them in the bathtub unattended," Dana said, "and as I was thinking of going into the bedroom to make a quick phone call, it did cross my mind that this was something I shouldn't do. But then I thought, 'It will only take a few minutes—nothing will happen.' The conversation lasted about 3 minutes.

"I could hear Laura playing and laughing, but I felt something was wrong. Something inside me said, 'Check on your kids.'" When Dana returned to the bathroom, she found Caroline out of her ring, floating belly up and no longer breathing. She pulled her from the water and frantically dialed 9-1-1.

"When I checked for her pulse, I couldn't find a heart rate," Dana said. "I thought I had let her drown." Dana's call reached dispatcher Stephanie Wyatt, who heard the desperate mother tell her, "My little girl fell in the tub—she's blue!"

Sheriff's Sergeant Jim Romine listened to Wyatt take the call, then left immediately to help. "When she said 'Your baby's blue?' I immediately thought of a dead baby. There was one thing on my mind, and that was to get there. I didn't know if it was going to make a difference or not, but I was going to try."

Although Caroline's mother was a registered nurse, in her panic she could not remember her emergency training. "I was hysterical. Everything I knew as a nurse went out the window. I thought I had lost my child," she said.

For a moment, dispatcher Wyatt felt herself affected by Dana's panic. "I was scared to death. I wasn't prepared mentally for the call," she said. "I had to control myself because I felt myself reacting as a mother, not as a dispatcher," she said. But she did gain control of herself, and patiently talked Dana through rescue breathing and CPR for her stricken child. "Keep it up," she told her. "Keep it up. Just keep going until they get there and take over."

Within 3 minutes of Dana's call, volunteer emergency medical technician Holly Jones and her husband were at Dana's house. "This was my first call as an EMT and it was extremely scary for me," Holly said. "You know, you think, 'Maybe I'm not ready for this.'" A city fire department unit also arrived, led by senior paramedic Chuck Hawman, and Dana hung up the phone, giving Caroline, who was barely breathing, over to his care. "My first thought was 'This kid's going to die,'" Hawman said. "There was absolutely no time to waste. We suctioned her airway really aggressively, and that was the turning point. We were able to suction out what was occluding her airway. That's when Caroline started to cry."

Back at the EMS center, Stephanie Wyatt had finally allowed herself to experience all the feelings she had suppressed while handling the call. "When the call is over, all the emotions that you put on the shelf just come flooding back into you. You just feel like you want to fall apart. I hoped and prayed that that baby would live—but I had no way of knowing," she said.

Sgt. Romine, who had also arrived at the scene of the emergency, did not forget Wyatt's concern, and called her to share the good news. "I heard the baby crying, and it sounded like gold," he said. "I got the phone, dialed the dispatcher, and said, 'Listen to this.'"

"I wasn't expecting that at all. We normally don't get that happening," Wyatt said. "I could have hugged him for doing that. Then I bawled my eyes out."

Caroline was not fully conscious when she arrived at St. Mary's Medical Center. "Typically, if the brain is deprived of oxygen for somewhere between 4 and 6 minutes, there is the potential of significant damage to the child," the physician who took charge of her case later said.

Dana and her husband, Doug, kept an anxious vigil at Caroline's bedside. "It was real hard because I just looked at her, and she was only 11 months old and superhelpless. It was so painful, just waiting for her to get up and say, 'Hey, let's go play.' It was like running in mud. You just didn't seem to be getting anywhere," Doug said.

"He sat next to her bed and talked to her for hours," Dana said. "It seemed like every hour she became more responsive, and by the morning she was sitting up and saying 'Daddy' and 'Mama.' It almost seemed like a miracle." Caroline was released from the hospital the next day, with no brain damage.

"When it happened, I felt terribly guilty. I felt, she has put her life in my hands and she's only a little person and I've failed her," Dana said. "I think I'm a good mom and I think I'm a good person, but I did something that was really irresponsible. If I can keep this from happening to one other person, it's worth it.

"The dispatcher played a huge role. I think she made the difference in saving Caroline's life. I can still remember her voice—it was very reassuring, like an angel."

"Drowning can occur in 1 inch of water, and the bathtub is the most likely place that a child will die or suffer a near-drowning. Caroline was very lucky," her doctor at the hospital said.

August 16, 1993, was a hot and sunny day in Burlington, Vermont. Fifteen-year-old Paula Haskell was inside her home, taking care of her three younger brothers. While David napped upstairs, Paula watched TV with 2-year-old Wesley and his 8-year-old brother, J. J. Paula and J. J. saw Wes wander out of the living room and heard him go upstairs, presumably to wake up David and coax him into playing.

A few minutes later, hearing no further sounds, Paula grew concerned and sent J. J. to look for Wes. He found him floating face up, unconscious, in the family swimming pool, and ran to get Paula, who began screaming in terror at the sight of her baby brother's motionless little body.

Donna Hayes, who was watching her three children playing in their pool next door, heard Paula's screams and sprang into action. "I knew something major had happened," Donna said. "She let out one long scream, and then she was completely hysterical. She just kept screaming and screaming and screaming."

Donna ran next door, and Paula told her, "Wesley's in the pool—he's drowned."

"Get him out," Donna said. Then she went back to her house, called 9-1-1, and rushed back next door to find Paula kneeling over Wes's body, rubbing his back. "I remember the smell of vomit and the purple—he was so purple, with these big white eyes," she said.

"I felt for a pulse, and didn't feel anything. I thought, 'Oh my God, how do you do CPR?' I gave him two rescue breaths, and then I knew his airway was open because his chest was beginning to rise. Then I went into chest compressions and then back to rescue breathing—and then I kept following the cycle. It was so hard—he was just so floppy and lifeless. I kept yelling, 'He's okay, Paula,' not knowing, of course, if he was, but just needing to calm her down."

"I was thinking, 'This is my fault. I'm supposed to be watching him and he's drowned because of me,'" Paula said.

For what seemed an unbearably long time, Wes did not appear to respond to Donna's efforts. "I have no idea how long I was doing it. It seemed like forever," Donna said. "Finally, I thought I saw his eyes move and he started to make noises. I knew then that something had happened—I knew his heart had started. Then I just kept doing rescue breathing, knowing that was not going to hurt him."

Within 5 minutes of Donna's call, she heard sirens at the front of her house and a rescue unit from the Burlington Fire Department arrived, which included EMT Brian Trudeau. "When we got there, the child was already breathing. He seemed to be conscious, but he wasn't really responding to us." Wes was rolled on his side to keep his airway clear until medics arrived to give him oxygen therapy, place him on a backboard as a precaution in case of spinal injury, and transport him to the nearest hospital.

"Donna reacted as calmly as anyone probably could," Trudeau said later, assessing the situation. "I think there's a very good chance that the child could have suffered some kind of brain damage had she not started the CPR."

"I never thought I'd be able to handle an emergency," Donna said, "but the fact that I knew CPR made me calm. Before we got our pool, I wanted my husband to be certified in CPR. He said, 'I've seen it on TV. I could probably do it.' I said, 'No, you need to know the details. You have to take a course.'"

Wesley was released from the hospital on the following day with no sign of permanent injury, to the enormous relief of his family. "The day after he came home, he was running around again and just fine," Paula said. "I can't express how thankful I am for everyone who helped. I've learned from this that you never take your eye off a child for a minute. You have no idea where a child can wander off to."

Bob Haskell, Wesley's father, put a fence around their pool the following week. "It doesn't take long to drown," he said. "I'm just so grateful that Donna was there. If she hadn't been, I think my son would be dead."

"It didn't really hit me until I saw Wes again," Donna said. "That was when I finally realized what had happened—that I had looked at a baby that had no life in him and given him the breath of life. It's incredible."

Treatment for Drowning If the Victim Is Not Breathing:

1. Call EMS personnel.
2. *Open the airway.* To do this, place the victim on a hard, flat surface (for an infant, this may be the palm of your hand). Kneel at the victim's side with your knee nearer the victim's head opposite his shoulders.

Always assume a head or neck injury in a drowning incident. First, try to open the airway by lifting the chin without tilting the head. If this doesn't work, use a modified jaw thrust:

a. Kneel at the top of the victim's head, leaning on your elbows.
b. Reach forward and gently place one hand on each side of the victim's chin, at the angles of the lower jaw.

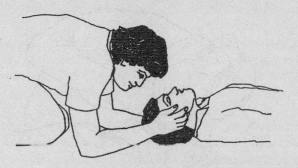

Modified Jaw-Thrust

   c. Push the victim's jaw forward, applying most of the pressure with your index fingers. Do not tilt or rotate the victim's head.

3. Check for breathing. See if the chest is rising and falling, listen for the sound of air escaping upon exhalation, and put your hand near the nostrils and mouth to feel for the flow of air.

4. If breathing has stopped, administer **rescue breathing** (artificial ventilation) by taking the following steps:

   a. Gently pinch the victim's nostrils shut with the thumb and index finger of the hand that is on his or her forehead.

   b. Take a deep breath and make a tight seal around the victim's mouth (nose and mouth for an infant or small child) with your mouth. Give two full breaths into the air passage(s), each one lasting about 1½ seconds, with a pause in between to let the air flow back out.

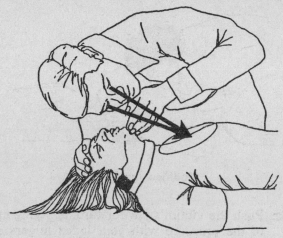

Establishing Breathlessness

Watch for the chest to rise after each breath to be certain that the air is going in. If the chest does not move, the airway may still be blocked, and you may have to tilt the head back farther.

c. Check for carotid pulse. If the victim has no pulse, administer CPR (see p. 229).

d. If the victim has a pulse, continue to breathe into his or her air passage at the rate of one breath every 5 seconds for an adult, every 4 seconds for a small child, and every 3 seconds for an infant (puffing the air in gently from the mouth). For an adult, breaths can be timed by counting "1-1,000, 2-1,000, 3-1,000," then taking a breath and exhaling slowly into the victim.

e. Each time, after exhaling into the victim's air

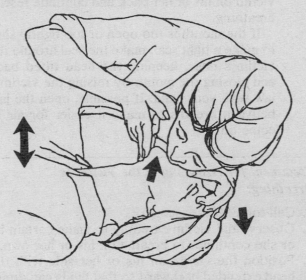

Two Breaths

passage, remove your mouth and turn your head to the side so that your ear is over his or her mouth, you can listen for his or her exhaling and watch the motion of his or her chest. Check for a pulse every minute (after every 12 breaths). If the victim's pulse fails, administer CPR. Continue until victim starts to breathe on his or her own, keeping the victim's head extended at all times.

If the victim starts to vomit, turn the head and body together, as a unit, so that the victim is lying on his or her side, to keep the vomit from entering the lungs. Then reposition the victim on his or her back and continue rescue breathing.

If the mouth is too open or too tightly shut to make a tight seal, make the seal around the victim's nose, keeping the head tilted back and closing the mouth by raising the victim's jaw with your hand. If possible, open the jaw between breaths to make it easier for air to come out.

Treatment for Drowning If the Victim Is Breathing:

1. Call for EMS assistance.
2. Observe the victim carefully to make certain he or she continues to breathe on his or her own.
3. Position the victim on his or her side with the head extended backward so that fluids can drain.
4. Keep the victim warm.
5. Reassure and comfort the victim.
6. Watch for signs of shock and treat for shock if necessary (see p. 305).
7. Do *not* give the victim food, water, or alcohol.

Shallow-Water Blackout

Shallow-water blackout can result in drowning if not caught in time. The victim (often a child) hyperventilates (takes in a large amount of air) in order to stay under water for an extended period of time. This lowers the carbon dioxide level in the blood below the point that stimulates the normal impulse to breathe. The victim can pass out while underwater owing to the lack of oxygen.

Blackout may have occurred if the victim has been underwater or lying face down in the water for longer than usual, or appears to be lifeless in the water.

Treat as for drowning, performing rescue breathing and CPR if necessary. Call EMS personnel or take the victim to the nearest hospital emergency room for further observation.

Water Rescue

It is important not to endanger yourself while attempting to rescue a drowning victim. If the victim is near the side of a pool, lie prone and give the victim your hand or foot, and pull him or her out. If the victim is too far away to reach in this way, reach out to him or her with a life preserver ring, pole, stick, board, rope, or other object. If he or she is near the shallow end of the pool, you can also wade in and pull him or her out. If the water is too deep to stand in securely but there is a pool ladder, overflow trough, piling, or other secure object you can grasp, enter the water and, holding onto this object, extend a hand or a foot to the victim.

If there is a chance that the victim has a head or spine injury, as in a diving accident, the victim's neck must be supported and kept in alignment with the body. This can be done by putting a board (a table leaf can be used for this purpose) under the victim's head and back while he or she is still in the water. The purpose is to keep the victim from moving and thus further injuring the spine. Lift the victim out of the water with the board.

If there is no board available, carefully tow or

push the victim into shallow water, grasping the armpits or legs, so that the motion is in the direction of the length of the body, keeping the head aligned with the body. If the victim is prone in the water, gently turn him or her on his or her back, keeping the head, neck, and trunk in alignment, supporting them and turning them as a unit. *Any* movement of the head, in any direction, can cause paralysis or death.

Water Safety and Drowning Prevention:

- Supervise young children when they are around water—any source of water. Do not take your eyes off them for a moment. They can drown in water that is only 1 inch deep.
- Do not rely on flotation devices to keep your child safe in the water. They can give a false sense of security.
- Never leave a child unattended in the bathtub. Do not answer the telephone or the door. Have everything that you need nearby.
- Keep the toilet lid closed to prevent accidental drowning of children and pets. Install a safety lock to keep the lid down.
- Keep buckets out of the reach of children. Each year, many children drown in buckets that have only a few inches of water in them.
- Enroll your children in a swimming and water safety class.
- Do not swim or dive alone.
- If you have long hair, tie it back or wear a bathing cap when you swim or engage in water

sports, so it doesn't get caught under water or tangled in equipment.

- Do not engage in horseplay in or around the swimming pool: don't run, jump into the water on top of others, dunk, or push.
- Do not dive head first into any water unless you have ascertained for yourself that it is deep enough.
- Secure swimming pools and hot tubs behind a safe fence with a secure gate.
- Make certain swimming-pool drains have secure drain covers. An open drain is inviting to children, and the force of suction in the drain can trap a finger and lead to drowning.
- Post emergency phone numbers and a CPR chart in a visible place by your swimming pool.
- Don't drink alcohol if you are planning to swim, dive, or play in a swimming pool.
- Don't drink alcohol in a hot tub, jacuzzi, or bathtub.
- Learn to perform rescue breathing on adults and infants.

Ear Injuries

Bleeding from the outside of the ear (the soft tissue) can be controlled by direct pressure.

Internally, the ear can be injured and the eardrum ruptured by a loud blast, a blow to the head, a fall, sudden pressure changes such as those caused by an explosion or a deep-water dive, or an object poked into the ear. The victim of such an injury may experience inner ear pain or loss of hearing or balance, and should seek professional medical treatment.

A serious head or spine injury may result in the presence of blood or other fluid in the ear canal or draining from the ear. If this is the case:

- Do *not* put anything in the ear.
- Do *not* attempt to control the flow of liquid by direct pressure or any other means.
- Loosely cover the ear with a bandage or a cloth to absorb the liquid.
- Place the victim on his or her injured side so that the affected ear is downward, facilitating drainage.

Foreign Objects in the Ear

Small insects, pieces of rock, or other material may become lodged in the ear. Children sometimes put objects in their ears, such as kernels of corn, peas, buttons, seeds, beans, beads, paper, and cotton. Some objects, such as seeds, absorb moisture once they are in the ear, swell in size, and become difficult to remove, sometimes causing infection.

Do *not* insert pins, match sticks, pieces of wire, or any other objects inside the ear to dislodge the foreign object. This can damage the tissue lining the ear or puncture the eardrum. Seek medical attention to remove any object lodged in the ear with the following exceptions:

- If a live insect is inside the ear, put several drops of warm oil (baby oil, mineral oil, or vegetable oil) inside the ear to kill the insect. Let the oil run out. If the insect does not come out with the oil, do not attempt to remove it. Seek medical attention.
- If a piece of paper or cotton lodged in the ear is clearly visible outside the ear canal, you may attempt to remove it with a pair of tweezers.

Electrical Injuries

Any electric current can be dangerous. Because of its high water content, the human body is a good conductor of electricity, which means that if you come in contact with an electrical current, it will pass through your body easily. Contact can come through an exposed power line, a malfunctioning electrical appliance, or lightning.

Lightning, which can carry up to 5,000,000 volts of electricity, causes more deaths annually in the United States than any other weather hazard, including blizzards, hurricanes, floods, tornadoes, and earthquakes. Every year, nearly 100 people are killed and about another 300 injured by lightning strikes.

Some parts of the body, such as the skin, resist the electrical current, producing heat, which can cause burns (see also burns, p. 67). These will occur at both the entrance site and the exit site of the current, and may cause deep, serious injury to underlying tissue in spite of the superficial appearance of the wounds. More seriously, electricity can cause paralysis of the nerve centers that control

171

breathing and stop or alter the regular beat of the heart. The amount of damage done depends on the type, amount, and duration of contact and the current's path through the body. Suspect an electrical injury if you hear a loud bang or pop and/or see an unexpected flash.

In August 1991, Connie and John Allen of Cincinnati, Ohio, who were excitedly expecting the birth of twins, had an unexpected encounter with electricity that almost left their unborn babies fatherless.

"It was Saturday afternoon, and we were having company the next day, and I wanted the yard to look beautiful," Connie said, "so I asked John to trim the hedges. They were old hedge trimmers, and they were falling apart, but they still worked, so he thought he'd just use them real fast." Because the three-pronged grounding plug on the trimmers was a little wobbly, John connected it to a two-pronged adapter, plugged the adapter into a power source and started to work on the hedges, which grew along a metal chain-link fence. Things went smoothly until John reached for the fence for support, and a powerful electric current shot through his body, leaving him rigid and erect, even after his hold on the trimmers and the fence had released.

"All of a sudden I heard a groan," said Connie, who had been sweeping leaves in the yard. "So I ran over and I touched his back, and he just kind of fell over. I called his name, but he wouldn't respond. His lips were turning blue, and I thought, 'He's dead. But how did he die?' I almost wanted to think that it was a joke, but I knew that he wasn't going to wake up. I had taken CPR before, but I was so distracted that I couldn't even think of following the correct steps." Connie did manage to give her husband artificial respiration, but to no avail. "So I decided that if I screamed as loud as I could, maybe somebody would hear."

"Help!" Connie yelled. "Please help us!"

Julia Krienbaum, a neighbor, heard Connie's cries and called 9-1-1. Reed Bogart, another neighbor, who lived two doors away, also heard Connie screaming and rushed over to help.

"It was very scary," Bogart said. "He's lying there and he's blue. I assumed he's dead, and I didn't even know why he was lying there. I didn't know CPR, but I gave him mouth-to-mouth resuscitation, hoping that I could do something."

"Is it working?" Connie asked desperately.

"No, it's not," Bogart told her.

"When I was pregnant, we were so excited to be having a baby," Connie said. "And then we found out it was twins, and he was ecstatic. [They were] going to be the light of John's life. That's all he could talk about. And here I realized that he could easily never see them."

Neighbors Lois Siegle, a registered nurse, and Sharon Burns had also heard Connie and raced to the scene. "When we approached the backyard, we saw John lying on his back, and he looked terrible," Burns said. "He was so blue and so lifeless that I couldn't imagine anybody coming back from that point," Siegle said. The women took over from Bogart and started doing CPR.

"She's seven months' pregnant. This is a time a lot

of babies are born premature, especially twins," said Siegle. "And I'm thinking, 'She's going to go into labor if she doesn't calm down.'"

"They kept telling me, 'You can't get this upset. You have to think about the babies.' At that point, I only wanted to see John wake up. I didn't want those babies without John."

Within 8 minutes of the 9-1-1 call, Cincinnati Fire Department rescue units arrived on the scene, led by Captain Earl Menkhaus. "When I first saw the victim, he was basically clinically dead," said Menkhaus. "Even though CPR was being applied, there was apparently not much oxygen getting to the victim, because his face was extremely blue. So we immediately proceeded with hooking up the Heartstarter 1000, a semiautomatic defibrillator. This Heartstarter 1000 machine was put on loan to the city of Cincinnati as a test program, because it was believed that a lot of lives could be saved by getting this equipment to people who are on the scene first. This machine showed that he was in a ventricular fibrillation, in which the heart is like a bag of worms beating against itself, and there is no rhythm to it, so that the defibrillator called for a shock."

"I kept glancing at him, thinking, 'He's just not coming around, and he should be by now,'" Siegle said.

Then one of the paramedics monitoring John's condition said the magic words: "I got a pulse, guys!"

"Okay, let's get him some oxygen," another paramedic said.

"When they turned around and said he was breathing on his own, it was like Christmas in July. It was the most wonderful feeling," said Siegle. "And then you just started praying that everything worked out all right."

John was taken to Providence Hospital in a coma, where he was examined by emergency physician Daniel Franklin. "Although we knew that CPR had been administered early and that he had been defibrillated early, there was a chance that he would not come out of the coma," Franklin said.

"It was a long wait for somebody to tell me that John was going to be okay," Connie said. "But in the back of my mind, I was afraid that the response was going to be 'Sorry, Mrs. Allen. Sorry, there was nothing we could do for your husband.' It was such a scary feeling." Finally, she was led in to see her husband. "I kept trying to take his hand and put it onto my stomach and say to John, 'Feel that. Your daughters are in there. They need you. You have to wake up.' They thought that maybe if you gave him a loud yell with a familiar voice, he'd wake up. So all night long I had been yelling, 'John! John!' And this time I yelled, 'John!' and he just sat up and turned his head from side to side and he just smiled." John had been in the coma for 20 hours.

The heart failure John suffered when he was electrocuted left him with no permanent damage. "I feel really lucky," John said. "This year alone, I've been blessed with twins and recovered from a near-fatal accident. I'm the luckiest guy in the world."

"There's not a day that goes by when I see John with the babies and I don't think, 'They could have been without this,'" Connie said. "I'm so grateful. I'm so happy for them that they get to have a daddy like John."

When the accident was investigated, it was discovered that the improperly grounded, frayed hedge trimmer cord was responsible for John's electrocution when he touched the metal fence. "Had that two-pronged adapter not been on the plug when he got the shock, the trimmers would have immediately turned off," Connie said. "When John was in his coma, I was promising him that he could play golf whenever he wanted, and that he would never have to do yard work again."

"She lied," John said, laughing. "It's funny, because your perspective changes so dramatically when something like this happens. You really focus on the important things in life, like your family and your kids. And that's what's important to me."

"I'm so grateful to Reed and Sharon and Lois, and that rescue squad," Connie said. "They saved John's life, and that means everything to us. So therefore they mean everything to us."

 On September 5, 1991, Lynn and John Endicott of Lakeside, California, also had a near-fatal encounter with electricity, but in their case, it came from the sky.

The Endicotts, who had rarely been able to get away together during their 7 years of marriage, had just returned from their first vacation in 3 years—an experience that they both believed had restored the intimacy of their relationship. "We had just come back from a camping trip," Lynn said. "Until then we really hadn't had a vacation or any time off together for a long time. It just put our relationship right back where it was when we first met. It was a very wonderful feeling for the two of us."

Lynn was preparing their first dinner at home after coming back when John, hearing their two dogs bark, decided to take them for a walk. "Hurry up," Lynn told him. "Dinner's ready."

"I'll just be a second, honey," John called out as he headed out of the door. About 15 seconds later, Lynn heard a deafening crash of thunder, which was accompanied by a brilliant flash of lightning.

"I was absolutely terrified," Lynn said. "I knew that lightning was close, and I knew he was out there." Lynn raced out into the pouring rain, and found her husband lying face down in the wet driveway, apparently struck by the lightning. "Johnny! Johnny!" she called, but there was no response. "There was absolutely nothing," she said, "nothing, nothing."

She ran back to the house and dialed 9-1-1. "Fire and medical emergency," said Heartland Communications Facility Authority dispatcher Scott Cullen, who took the call. He took Lynn's address and immediately dispatched Lakeside Fire Department medics to the scene. Then he proceeded to get more information from Lynn about her husband's condition.

"He's just lying in our front yard," she said.

"Okay, is he conscious?"

"No, he's not."

"Is he breathing?"

"No. Please, what do I do now?" Lynn asked desperately.

"Okay, they're on their way. They'll be right there, okay?" Cullen said.

"You've got to help me. What can I do?" Lynn pleaded.

"I knew right away from the emotional level that

it was something pretty serious," Cullen said. "Can you bring the phone out where he is?" he asked Lynn.

"Yes, I can," she said, although in reality the phone extension nearest to where John was lying was in the garage, a good distance from where his body lay sprawled. "You've got to help me," she repeated.

"I started to hesitate about giving CPR instructions, because, technically, I hadn't been told that I could do this," said Cullen, who had fortuitously completed an emergency medical dispatch course just 2 hours before the call came in. Legally, he was not yet allowed to give medical instructions, and the conflicted dispatcher tried once more to reassure Lynn. "The medics are on their way now," he told her. "They'll be there in a short period of time. Is he breathing?" he asked Lynn again.

"No."

"Is there any way you can get him to near where the phone is?"

"Can I drag him?"

"Can you drag him close enough? They're already on their way. I'm just staying on the phone with you."

"I knew that we had to get him near the phone," Cullen later said, "and it was totally up to her to do it."

"I grabbed him and I tried to drag him to the garage, but he was too heavy," Lynn said. "My first thought was that I was going to spend the rest of my life alone without him, and I couldn't do that. I don't know how, but I just got the strength somewhere down inside of me, got ahold of him, and dragged him however many feet it was to the garage." When she had gotten her husband's 180-pound body to the edge of the garage, she returned to the phone. "You've got to help me," she said again to Cullen.

"Okay, is he by where you're at?" Cullen asked.

"Yes."

"Okay, I want you to shake his shoulders and yell at him—make sure he's unconscious. Do it now," he told her. "The initial objective before you give anybody CPR is to make sure they are not conscious, that they do not have a pulse, and that they are not breathing," he later explained, "because you can hurt someone if they don't need CPR."

"Did he respond at all?" he asked Lynn.

"No."

"Is he breathing?"

"No."

"Are you sure?"

"Positive," she said.

"The engine is going to be there any minute," Cullen said, still hoping that he would not have to give her the instructions he was legally bound to withhold.

"No," Lynn said emphatically, "I can't see them coming over the hill. They're not here. Help me now!"

"If you lose your job for doing the right thing, then you lose your job," Cullen later said of his decision. "There's a moral imperative here. If I don't tell her what to do, he's going to die. No question about it."

Now Cullen told Lynn, "I want you to go kneel on the side of your husband next to his head. I want you to place the palm of your hand that's closest to his feet under his neck and use your other hand to push his head back and tilt his head back. Do it now." Cullen was giving her the instructions for opening John's airway and checking for breathing, the first step before starting CPR.

"As soon as I was on my way back to John, I knew what the answer was already," Lynn said. "I knew there was nothing there."

"He's still not breathing?" Cullen asked her when she returned to the phone.

"No," she said desperately.

"Now calm down, we're going to get through this," Cullen told her, and proceeded to instruct her in giving John the two rescue breaths that begin the CPR cycle of pulmonary and cardiac assistance. "Blow into his mouth and see if his chest rises."

"It rises. It's making a gurgling noise," Lynn said. Cullen then instructed her how to feel for John's pulse on the side of his neck. "There's no pulse," Lynn reported.

"The medics are going to be there," he said, trying to encourage her, and proceeded to instruct her in giving John chest compressions. "I was very nervous," Cullen said, "because he was basically clinically dead."

After the 15 compressions, Cullen told her to go back to the rescue breathing.

"He's just blurting it out," Lynn said, discouraged.

"Is he breathing?"

"No."

"Okay, I want you to keep doing that—the breathing and then the compressions—until the paramedics get there," Cullen told her.

"One, two, three, four, five, six, seven—God—eight, nine . . ." Lynn panted, counting the compressions.

"You're doing fine," Cullen encouraged her.

"The more I did the compressions, the more frustrated I got," Lynn said. "There was no response from John at all—nothing."

"One, two, three, help me, five—help me—seven . . ." Lynn went on.

"Keep going, you're doing fine."

". . . eight, nine—don't die! don't die!—eleven, twelve—I love him—fourteen."

"Okay, just stay calm. Just keep doing what you're doing. You're helping him," Cullen said. "With a full arrest, you start CPR and you don't stop until somebody comes in and takes over," he explained later. "We have to make them understand that they are helping by doing what they're doing."

"Tell them to come quicker," Lynn yelled, finishing another compression count.

"They're on their way," Cullen said again.

"They're right here," she said excitedly, almost as soon as the words were out of his mouth.

It was 12 minutes since Cullen had first picked up the phone to take Lynn's call, and paramedics from the Lakeside Fire Department were on the scene, including Scott Culkin, who was on his first call as a paramedic. "My initial concern was still lightning striking in the area," Culkin said. "My first concern was to get the patient quickly loaded into the ambulance. The patient was in a rhythm called asystole, which is also known as a flat line on the monitor. The patient was clinically dead."

"I asked them at the time, 'Were you able to start his heart on its own?' and they said, 'No,'" Lynn said. "It didn't look very good, but somehow I just couldn't give up. He wouldn't give up on me and I would never give up on him. Ever."

"We gave the patient several rounds of medication, and we got no response," said Culkin. "At that point, we felt that the patient probably would not survive. He remained on a flat line with no pulses and never was breathing on his own." Thirty minutes after

John's heart had stopped beating and 2 minutes before the ambulance arrived at the emergency department at Valley Medical Center, the paramedics received an order by radio phone from their base hospital physician to give John sodium bicarbonate, which was a deviation from their standard protocol for cardiac arrest. "Apparently, the base hospital physician knew what lightning did to the heart," Culkin said, "but I don't think that any of us felt that he would survive this, although he did have a pulse when we delivered him."

Thirty-five-year-old John Endicott was taken to the University of California San Diego Medical Center and put under the care of Dr. David Hoyt. "John was in a deep coma," Hoyt said. "His CT [computed tonography] scan suggested that his injury was due to the fact that he had had a cardiac arrest. His EEG [electroencephalogram] also suggested that he was not likely to make any useful recovery."

"A doctor finally came out after they had worked on him for over an hour," Lynn said. "The first thing he did was he gave me my husband's wedding ring, and then he started to tell me that things were not very good."

"We tried everything," the doctor told her.

"Somehow I felt that he was talking to someone else, but he was looking at me in the eyes, saying, 'Your husband's going to die.'"

In spite of the grim prognosis, Lynn did not give in to despair, and visited John for hours every day, even though he was comatose. "I would go in and talk to him or hold his hand. I always touched him and I was always talking to him and telling him what was going on; that I missed him and loved him. I used to sing to him, 'Johnny Angel, Johnny Angel.' But I never gave up hope."

"We try hard to balance what we call hope with the concern that we don't want to prolong unnecessary suffering," said Hoyt. "What we did with his wife is talk to her, to allow her to participate in the decision as to whether we should continue support or consider backing off."

"They were talking about *if* he lived, he had a 1% chance of becoming a functioning human being," Lynn said. "That's like somebody who can get out of bed, and that's about it. Has no thought process at all." But after 2 weeks, amazingly, Lynn did see a change in her husband's condition. "I just walked right over to him and leaned right down to him and gave him a kiss right on the lips, and he kissed me back. So I did it a second time, just to be sure that I wasn't imagining things. And he kissed me back, a second time. That's when I knew that there was someone in there and he knew who I was."

Five weeks after being struck by lightning, John was released from the hospital, but it took 20 months of speech, physical, and occupational therapy before he could return to work. "I'm happy to be alive. I want to thank everyone who saved my life," John said. "Without their help, I wouldn't be here today. I hope that someday I can repay them."

"He's got short-term memory problems right now and sometimes his reactions are a little slower than they used to be," said Lynn, "but physically there are no scars or any other problems. He's just not quite as strong as he used to be, but in time that will come back. It truly is a miracle that he is alive."

"The most amazing thing to me about John's recovery is that fact that we were wrong," said Hoyt. "We had lost hope, but his wife did not. She saw us through that extra week and that made the difference. I think there's no question that had she lost hope at that point, there might have been a different outcome."

"It's wonderful to have him back," Lynn said. "We'd like to go on someday and maybe even have a family. And we're just so glad to be back together. Scott Cullen, the emergency operator, didn't just do what he had to do. He made a judgment on his own to give me that CPR information, and my husband is alive because he made that decision. I could never tell him thank you enough."

"I've been a dispatcher for 9 years," Cullen later testified in 1993, "and this last year is the first year that they've let us give these prearrival instructions. A lot of people are under the impression that when they call 9-1-1, the people on the other end are going to be able to tell them exactly what to do—CPR mouth-to-mouth, whatever. But the sad fact is that most fire departments do not allow dispatchers to tell them what to do. There's nothing more helpless than a dispatcher when somebody calls up and says, 'What do I do? What do I do?' and you have to sit there and say, 'Well, I can't tell you what to do' because the agency you work for is worried about getting sued by somebody.

"It's a call that I'll never forget. It was my first CPR, and John survived. And I really thank the Lord that he's around."

Signs and Symptoms of Electrical Injury:

➤ Unconsciousness
➤ Dazed, confused behavior
➤ Obvious burns on the skin surface
➤ Weak, irregular, or absent pulse
➤ Weak, shallow, or virtually undetectable breathing
➤ Burns where the current both entered and exited, often on the hand or foot

Treatment for Electrical Injuries:

1. If the victim is free from contact with the electrical current (as is always the case with lightning), activate EMS if necessary and then begin first aid at once. If the victim is still in contact with the current, do *not* touch him or her until the current has been turned off or the victim is no longer in contact with it. Otherwise, you may risk electrocution yourself.

2. If the victim is in contact with the current, act as quickly as possible to remove the victim from contact with the current or the current from contact with the victim, since every second of delay reduces the possibility of resuscitation. Turn off the electrical current by removing the fuse or pulling the main switch. If this is not possible or if the victim is outside, have someone call the electric company to cut off the electricity.

3. Push the victim away from the wire with a non-conducting *dry* board, stick, or broom handle, or pull the victim away with a *dry* rope looped around the victim's arm or leg. *Never* use any-

thing metallic, wet, or damp. Do not touch the
victim until he or she is free from the wire.

4. Call EMS personnel.
5. If the victim has been struck by lightning, there
may be spinal injuries as well, so do not move
him or her unless absolutely necessary.
6. Maintain an open airway. Restore breathing and
circulation if necessary (see pp. 160 and 229).
7. Cover any burn injuries with a dry, sterile
dressing.
8. Treat for shock (see p. 305).

Tips for Preventing Electrical Injuries:

- Turn the light off before changing a light bulb.
Don't use a higher-watt bulb than the lamp can
safely handle.
- Make certain all your electrical appliances are
properly grounded.
- When unplugging an electrical appliance, always pull from the plug, not from the wire.
- Cover all exposed, unused wall outlets with
safety plugs.
- Teach your children never to put anything in
an electrical outlet.
- Keep all electrical appliances and the cords
attached to the appliances out of the reach and
climbing range of children.
- Replace old, damaged extension cords.
- Teach your children that if their kite becomes
tangled in power lines, release the string at
once and don't try to remove it.
- Stay well away from any downed power line.
- Lightning is attracted to metal, water, and any-

thing tall. If you are indoors when a lightning storm strikes, stay away from the fireplace, open windows, and doors. Also avoid water, stay off the phone, and unplug the television and the computer.

- To reduce the risk of being struck by lightning if you are caught outdoors in a storm, avoid hilltops, tall trees, telephone poles, open fields, bodies of water, evergreens, metal objects (including small metal vehicles, such as motorcycles, bicycles, farm equipment, and golf carts), or isolated sheds. Go inside a large building or home if you can, or go into a car and roll up the windows. In an open field, kneel or squat in order to minimize contact points with the ground. Do not lie flat. If you are in a group, stay several yards apart.
- If you are swimming or boating, get out of the water as soon as you see or hear a storm.

Eye Injuries

Blunt Injuries to the Eye (Black Eye)

An injury to the eye from a hard blow like that from a moving ball or a fist requires medical attention by an ophthalmologist or an emergency-department attending physician, even though it may not look serious, because of the possibility of internal bleeding in the eye.

Treatment for Black Eye:

1. Apply cold compresses to the injured eye.
2. Have the victim lie down with both eyes closed.

Cuts to the Eye

Any cut to the eye, including the eyelid, can be extremely dangerous and result in blindness if immediate action is not taken.

Treatment for Cuts to the Eye:

1. Cover the injured eye with a sterile pad or gauze, or a clean, folded cloth, and bandage in place,

but apply no pressure. Also cover the uninjured eye to prevent eyeball movement.

2. Seek medical care immediately, preferably from a physician who is an eye specialist or at the nearest hospital emergency room. If possible, the victim should be transported while he or she is lying down.

Injuries Caused by Objects in the Eye

Treatment for Objects Impaled in the Eye:

1. Call EMS personnel if necessary, or arrange to transport the victim, who should be lying on his or her back if possible, to a medical facility. While waiting for EMS to arrive, or before transporting the victim:
2. Do *not* attempt to remove the object from the eye.
3. Place the victim on his or her back.
4. Place a sterile dressing around the object.
5. Stabilize the object in place. You can use a paper cup to support the object.
6. Carefully bandage the cup in place.
7. Apply a bandage covering both eyes.

Treatment for Objects Embedded in the Eyeball:

1. If you suspect there is an object embedded in the eyeball, do not allow the victim to rub his or her eyes.
2. Before examining the eyeball to search for the object, wash both hands with soap and water.

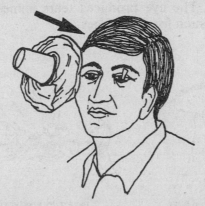

Dressing for an Embedded Object in the Eye

3. Do not attempt to remove the object from the eyeball.
4. Gently cover both eyes with sterile or clean bandages (to keep the eyes from moving) and bandage gently in place.
5. Seek medical attention promptly, preferably from an eye specialist or a hospital emergency room. If possible, the victim should be transported while he or she is lying down on his or her back.

Particles such as dirt, cinders, sand, or slivers of wood or metal frequently enter the eye and lodge there, floating on the eyeball or inside the eyelid. They can cause discomfort, inflammation, and possibly infection. The victim may have difficulty opening the eye because light further increases the irritation. The eye produces tears immediately to flush out such foreign bodies.

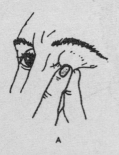
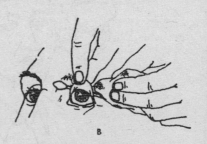

A
PULL UPPER EYELID OVER
LOWER EYELASHES

B
LIFT EYELID, REMOVE OBJECT
WITH STERILE GAUZE

Removal of a Foreign Body on the Inside of the Eyelid

Treatment for Foreign Bodies in the Eye but Not Embedded in the Eyeball:

1. Do not allow the victim to rub his or her eyes, which might scratch the eyeball or cause the object to become embedded in it.
2. Tell the victim to blink several times to try to dislodge the object.
3. Gently bring the upper lid down over the lower lid and hold it there for a moment, then release it. This produces more tears, which may wash the object away. Or, if the object is lodged under the upper lid, its undersurfaces will be drawn over the lashes of the lower lid and the object may be removed in this way.
4. Step 3 may cause an object to be deposited on

the eyeball from the upper lid. If this is the case, or if the object is already on the surface of the eyelid, gently flush the eye with water, using a medicine dropper, a glass, or holding the victim's head under a gentle stream of water, or:

5. Lifting the upper lid, gently remove the object from the eyeball with a piece of sterile gauze.

6. If the object does not appear to be on the eyeball, but irritation is still felt, pull down the lower lid and, if it is seen there, gently remove it with the moistened corner of a clean handkerchief, cloth, or facial tissue.

7. If the object is not seen in the lower lid, ask the victim to look down, and while he or she is doing so, raise the upper lid and look for it there. If it is seen there, hold the eyelid down and place the end of a cotton swab, a kitchen match, or similar object across the back of the lid and flip the lid backward over it. With the victim still looking down, remove the object from the lid with the moistened end of a clean handkerchief, tissue, or cloth.

8. If the object still remains, have the victim seek medical attention.

Fainting

Fainting is a sudden and temporary partial or complete loss of consciousness due to an inadequate supply of oxygen to the brain. The reduced blood flow to the brain that causes this can come from the blood pooling in the legs and lower body. Fainting can be triggered by the sight of blood or other emotional shocks. It can also be caused by pain, specific medical conditions such as heart disease, weakness or exhaustion (as from standing for a long period of time or from overexertion), heat, or, among certain people (such as pregnant women and the elderly), from suddenly changing positions, as in going from sitting to standing up.

Signs and Symptoms of Fainting (Any or All May Be Present):

➤ Fainting may occur with or without warning. Initially, the victim may feel weak and dizzy, and may see spots.
➤ The face becomes pale and the lips blue.
➤ The forehead is covered with cold perspiration.

➤ The skin is pale, cool, and moist.
➤ The victim is nauseated.
➤ There is numbness and weakness in the fingers and toes.
➤ The pulse is rapid and weak.
➤ Breathing is shallow.

Fainting usually resolves itself. When the victim collapses, normal blood flow to the brain resumes and he or she usually regains consciousness within 1 minute.

Treatment for Fainting:

1. If a person feels faint, have him or her sit and slowly bend over until his or her head is between the knees, and hold that position. Alternatively, have the person lie down with legs elevated 8 to 12 inches.
2. If the person starts to collapse and you can reach him or her, lower him or her to the ground or other flat surface and position the person on his or her back. Then elevate the legs.
3. Loosen any restrictive clothing around the person's neck or waist.
4. If the victim vomits, place him or her on his or her side or turn the head to the side to prevent choking.
5. Do *not* give the victim anything to eat or drink.
6. Do *not* pour water on the victim's face.
7. Gently bathe the victim's face with cool water.
8. If the victim does not seem to recover com-

pletely or remains unconscious for any length of time, call EMS personnel or transport the victim to a medical facility. Check for airway, breathing, and circulation, and administer rescue breathing (see p. 161) and/or CPR (see p. 229) accordingly.

Head, Neck, and Spinal Injuries

Injuries of the head, neck, and spine, which often damage both bone and soft tissue, account for a small percentage of all injuries but for more than half of all fatalities in the United States every year. Since it is often difficult to assess the extent of damage caused by these injuries without x-rays it is advisable to provide first-aid treatment as if the injury is serious. While more head and spinal column injuries occur as the result of motor vehicle accidents than any other cause, a large percentage happen as the result of accidents in and around the home, mostly from falls, diving mishaps, and other athletic activities. Any situation in which the victim has fallen from a height greater than his or her own, or is found unconscious for unknown reasons, is one in which the possibility of a head or spinal injury should be considered. Any injury that penetrates the head or trunk, such as a gunshot wound or impalement on a sharp object, such as a knife or scissors, could also result in serious damage to these areas.

Andrea Jones and Scott Burdette are two young

people who were lucky enough to survive severe head and spinal injuries, owing to the actions of those around them and superb emergency medical care. They both learned sobering lessons about the dangers of taking unnecessary risks through nearly tragic accidents which changed their lives.

In April 1992, 16-year-old Andrea Jones and her best friend, Rachel Koets of Grand Rapids, Michigan, went south with Andrea's family for the school spring break. On their last night at the condominium in Gulf Shores, Alabama, Andrea and Rachel decided to get around their midnight curfew and sneak out to meet some boys for a final late-night beach party.

After saying good night to Andrea's mother, Kathy, and pretending to go to bed, the two girls surreptitiously made their exit from the sixth-floor apartment by lowering themselves from balcony railing to balcony railing. Rachel, being the taller of the two, went first, to help ease Andrea's precarious drop. They both made it down to the fourth floor, and Rachel was safely on the third-floor balcony when Andrea's grip on the railing above was weakened by dew and she went plummeting past her friend, landing on her back on the concrete pool area, 25 feet below.

Rachel rushed downstairs while the people in the third-floor unit called 9-1-1. "Can you hear me? Can you hear me?" Rachel shouted to her motionless friend. "There was blood coming from behind her ear, and her eyes were bulging out of her head," Rachel said. "It was like a horror movie, right before my eyes, and I just couldn't believe it was real. I thought that she was dead, and all I could think about was our parents. How was I going to explain this—that we did this for a bunch of guys?"

Fortunately, witnesses at the scene knew enough not to move Andrea, and Rachel covered her with a blanket to help prevent shock. Within 5 minutes of the call, the Gulf Shores Fire and Rescue Department arrived, led by paramedic corporal Mitchel Sims. "In my experience with patients who have fallen, the outcome is usually very poor," Simms said. "Time is so critical with trauma victims. Because of the brain's swelling from injury, there can be irreversible brain damage."

Andrea's mother and father rushed down to the pool area as soon as they were notified about the accident. "Words can't describe what it's like to see your child suffering and in pain," Kathy Jones said. "All I kept thinking was 'Please, God, take care of her and keep her alive.'"

"Deep in my heart," said paramedic Simms, "I did not think that this girl was going to make it. I looked at one of the guys on the ambulance and told him that her mother's heart was probably going to be broken tonight."

Andrea was taken by Life Flight helicopter to Baptist Hospital in Pensacola, Florida, where a trauma team awaited her arrival. "Apparently, she landed right on her head," said James Luker, the emergency physician leading the team. "That kind of impact delivers a terrific force, and my first thought was 'This is a 16-year-old who won't go back home.'"

Emergency nurse Donna Russell was one of those also treating Andrea. "She was jerking her body in a way we call 'posturing,' which is indicative of brain

----

damage," Russell said. "Very rarely do people with this kind of injury survive, and in our hearts we thought she was going to die."

When Dr. Luker studied the X-rays and the CT scan, he was amazed to discover that the only injury Andrea had sustained was to her head. He was also discouraged, because the injury appeared to be quite severe. Over the next 12 hours, Andrea's condition deteriorated as her brain continued to swell. The pressure inside her skull was at 88 on a scale on which sustained readings above 30 predict mortality. Doctors decided to perform an unusual emergency procedure and remove part of Andrea's skull. "This was a last-ditch effort," Dr. Luker said. "The chances of survival in a person who has this degree of injury are very, very small."

Meanwhile, Andrea's mother continued to maintain her faith in her daughter's recovery. "I just kept thinking, 'Fix her up and I'll take her home,'" Kathy Jones said. Then one of the doctors came to ask Kathy the question they are required by law to ask the families of victims in whom brain death may be imminent. "I may come back to you at a later time," he said, "and ask you to give permission for your daughter's organs to be harvested."

"It wasn't until then that I realized how serious this was and that she could die," Kathy said.

After the operation to relieve the pressure on her brain, Andrea was in a coma. "The question," Donna Russell said, "was if she did survive, what to do? We use an awfully harsh term in the medical profession—we call them vegetables. They lie there. You sprinkle them. You feed them. They grow. You hurt for the patient. You hurt for the family."

"We followed the nurse into Andrea's room," said Kathy Jones, speaking of her first visit to her daughter's bedside. "We saw her lying in bed, and she was perfectly still. All I could think was 'Please, recover so I can talk to you again.'"

A week later, on Good Friday, a nurse came to bring Andrea's parents what she described as "the best Easter gift they could have."

"We walked into her room," Kathy Jones said, "and she was sitting up in her chair. The week after, she was walking in the halls, joking with the nurses, complaining about the food."

In July the missing piece of Andrea's skull was replaced, and she proceeded with a rapid and complete recovery. One of the hardest things for both Andrea and Rachel, who was still haunted by guilt, was reconstructing their friendship. "Rachel feels very guilty," Andrea said, 6 months after the accident. "And sometimes she stays away a little bit."

"It's hard for me to deal with everything that happened," Rachel said. "We're not as close as we used to be. I wish that we were. I'd give everything that I own to have things back the way they were."

"I really want to be her friend so much again," Andrea said. "I think that she needs me as a friend again to let her know that I am okay. You should think before you do things, because you can hurt people who really do love you. You're hurting them and you're hurting yourself, and you're missing life."

"It's a super miracle that she's with us," said Jerry Jones, Andrea's father. "I want to thank the people who gave their prayers and best wishes to us—I want to thank them all."

"I would have bet a million dollars that she'd be

lying in bed for the rest of her life," said another one of Andrea's friends. "But to see her today, walking and talking and cheerleading, it's just wonderful."

"I'm very lucky to have my daughter back with me," said Kathy Jones. "Every day, I cherish the knowledge that I can see her, that I can talk to her, and that she is still part of our family."

On a hot day in May 1991, in the suburbs of Greenville, South Carolina, a close-knit group of friends from the local high-school band gathered at a backyard above-ground pool to try to cool off. Eighteen-year-old Scott Burdette and his 16-year-old girlfriend, Kelly Hart, who had been going together for almost a year, were there, fooling around in the 4½-foot-deep water, watching some of the boys jump off a bench that had been placed on the deck beside the pool.

"Some of the guys were having a contest," Kelly said, "doing cannonballs into the pool, and making up other kinds of dives. We were on the side, watching them goofball. Then Scott went up to do a dive."

Scott had planned to do a belly flop, but realizing that hitting the water this way could be painful, he changed his mind in midair and tried to bring his hands around in front of him to do a cannonball. Instead, he entered the pool head first, striking the bottom of the pool and causing a sudden trauma to his spine. Instantly paralyzed, he was unable to move anything below his neck. His motionless body floated to the surface, but at first nobody realized that anything was seriously the matter.

"I didn't think anything was wrong because he's

always joking around," Kelly said, "so nobody thought he was hurt." Scott's body sank to the bottom of the pool again, and when he resurfaced he started choking and calling for help. "I went over there and grabbed him by the waist," Kelly said. "He said that his neck was hurt. And then he said, 'Kelly, I can't move.' I was scared. Real scared."

Kelly called for Scott's sister, Krista, who was also in the pool. "I went over to where Kelly was holding him," Krista said, "and I put my hands on his back and said, 'Scott, are you really hurt?' because he plays around so much. And he said. 'Yeah, man, I'm really hurt—hurt serious.'"

Somebody yelled that they should get Scott out of the pool, but Kelly remembered what two EMS workers who had given a talk at their school had said. "They told us, 'Do not move the victim in case of head and spinal cord injuries. It could cause paralysis.'" Ignoring the urging of others to get Scott out of the water, she stabilized his head and emphatically told them not to touch him.

Some one inside the house called 9-1-1. Dispatcher Carolyn Northway took the call. "Right away, the caller told me that it was a diving accident, which led me to believe there was the possibility of paralysis," Northway said. "Uppermost in my mind was not to get him out of the pool until our trained personnel arrived to secure his neck and get him out without further damaging him." Rescue workers from the Berea Fire Department and the Greenville County EMS were dispatched to the scene.

"I started realizing that he was really hurt," Krista said, "and I kept shaking. We were trying to hold him really still, but I kept shaking."

"I was crying; I was shaking," said Kelly. "I was feeling that I was going to move him, and I knew that I had to keep calm, because if I moved, I could have hurt him very badly."

One of Scott's friends called his mother, Earlette Burdette. "I'm a nurse, and I know the things that happen when kids jump into a pool, so the first thing I did was say a prayer,"," she said. "Then I got in the car and went over there."

Off-duty paramedic Tom Kickler heard the report of the accident on the scanner and rushed over to see if he could help. "I took my shoes and socks off and eased myself into the water to try to reduce any effect of ripples because any movement might aggravate his injury. I asked him how he was doing. He was conscious and he said he wasn't having any trouble breathing, but he wasn't able to move any of his extremities, and at that point he had some numbness in his arms and legs."

When the medic unit arrived, EMS supervisor Bill Marcley took charge. Tom took over the task of immobilizing Scott's head, putting a cervical collar around his neck to keep him from moving it. "Once we had everybody assembled and had sufficient personnel in the pool to handle the situation," Marcley said, "we rotated Scott onto his back, being very careful to keep his head in line with his body. We put a backboard under him and secured him to it in such a way as to completely immobilize the body, from head to toe."

Scott's mother arrived just as the paramedics were ready to remove him from the pool. "I just went over to him and told him that I was there," she said. "I could see fear in his eyes, but he was very quiet. He didn't try to speak or anything."

"It was hurting to see my brother being taken away," said Krista. "I kept trying not to cry before, but then when we got on the deck, it just all started coming out."

"We had a friend whose brother-in-law had had a motor bike accident that paralyzed him," Scott's mother said. "Several months ago, Scott and I were talking and he said to me, 'Mom, if anything like that ever happens to me, I want you to pull the plug.' And that kind of means 'I don't want to live that way.'"

"I was thinking that he wasn't going to get to do the stuff that he wanted to do—go to college, get to do what he planned on doing," Kelly said. "And I wasn't sure what was going to happen between us."

Scott was transported to Greenville Memorial Hospital, where he was examined by neurosurgeon O. M. Ballenger. "The x-rays showed that he had a broken neck," Dr. Ballenger said. "If he were allowed to bend his neck forward another quarter of an inch at the scene of the accident, he probably would have been permanently paralyzed."

"Kelly deserves a lot of credit," said Tom Kickler. "She resisted the attempts and the pleas of other teenagers to remove Scott from the pool. If Kelly had done so, the outcome would have been tragically different, I'm certain.'"

Six months after Dr. Ballenger's operation, in which he successfully fused Scott's fractured vertebrae, Scott had made an amazing recovery.

"I really love Kelly a lot, and I really do appreciate her saving my life," Scott said. "There's not really words that you can say for stuff like that."

"He's always treated me nice," Kelly said, "but I think he does seem sweeter [now], at least to me. I was going to stay with him even if he was paralyzed.

And I think that was what was going through his mind, too—that he was scared that he was going to lose me also. But I was going to stick with him, no matter what happened."

"I feel closer to Kelly than anyone he's ever dated, just because I know that she cares about him, and I trust her more than I do anybody else," Krista said.

Kelly is grateful that she had the chance to learn first-aid techniques in school. "I think the lesson is pay attention to what you hear, because I had no idea as I was sitting there, listening to those EMS workers, that I was going to be using the procedures that I had learned," she said.

"I think that some teenagers at some time or another do learn the lesson of their own mortality," said Scott's mother.

"It made me realize that life can be taken away from you in a snap," Scott said. "I think it's made me grow up a little bit more. I think it's made the whole group grow up a little bit more."

Always call EMS personnel when a serious head or spine injury is suspected. The following signs and symptoms, while not always indicative of such injuries, may suggest them when combined with a knowledge of the cause of the injury. Be aware that they may not always appear immediately after the injury.

Signs and Symptoms of Injuries of the Head, Neck, or Spine:

➤ Unconsciousness
➤ Changes in the level of consciousness, such as drowsiness or confusion

➤ Severe pain or pressure in the head, neck, or back
➤ A cut, bruise, lump, or depression in the scalp or unusual bumps or depressions in the spine; bruising around the eyes or behind the ears
➤ Persistent headache
➤ Tingling or loss of sensation in the extremities
➤ Partial or complete loss of movement of any body part
➤ Blood or other fluids in the ears or nose or blood in the mouth
➤ Profuse external bleeding from the head, neck, or back
➤ Nausea or vomiting
➤ Impaired breathing or vision as a result of the injury
➤ Seizures or convulsions
➤ Dizziness or loss of balance
➤ Pupils of the eyes of unequal size
➤ Difficulty with speech
➤ Restlessness and/or confused behavior
➤ Change in the pulse rate

Injuries to the head, neck, and spine can become life-threatening emergencies. To reduce the possibilities of this happening, the following steps should always be taken, while awaiting the arrival of EMS personnel.

Treatment for Head, Neck, and Spinal Injuries:

1. Minimize movement of the head and spine. This is essential because excessive movement when there is an injury can do irreversible damage to

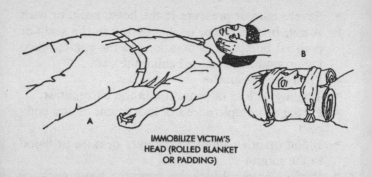

IMMOBILIZE VICTIM'S
HEAD (ROLLED BLANKET
OR PADDING)

Stabilizing the Head

the spinal cord. To minimize movement of the head and neck, a simple technique called *in-line stabilization* is used. To do this, place your hands on both sides of the victim's head, with your palms on his or her jaw if you are facing the victim, the base of his or her skull if you are behind the victim, or his or her temples if the victim is lying down and you are kneeling at his or her head. Gently position the head in line with the rest of the body, if it is not already in that position, and support it there until advanced medical care is available.

A broken neck can also be immobilized by wrapping a towel, sweater, newspaper, or some other soft item about 4 inches wide around the victim's neck, keeping the victim's head as still as possible. Folded towels, blankets, clothing, or other suitable objects, banked by bricks, sandbags, books, or other heavy objects may also be placed around the head, neck, and shoulders to keep the neck from moving.

Do *not* move the head to align with the body in the following cases:

- The victim's head is at an extreme angle to one side.
- The victim complains of pain, pressure, or muscle spasms when the head is initially moved.
- You feel resistance when trying to move the victim's head.

In these situations, support the victim's head in the position in which you find it.

2. Maintain an open airway. It is not necessary to roll the victim onto his or her back to check breathing, and, with injuries of this sort, to do so could be damaging. Look for chest movement and listen for the sound of breathing while maintaining in-line traction and immobilization of the head, neck, and spine at all times. If the victim is breathing, support him or her in the position in which you find him or her. If the victim begins to vomit, position him or her on one side to keep the airway clear. If this requires rolling the victim over, be careful to maintain in-line stabilization. *Always* ask someone to help you with this, if another person is available.

If the victim is not breathing and is not already on his or her back, roll the victim over gently, keeping his or her head in the same position in which it was found. Tilt his or her head backward only very slightly to provide and maintain an open airway, and give rescue breaths (see p. 161).

3. Monitor consciousness and breathing. This can

be done while stabilizing the head and neck. The victim may become incoherent or respond to questions inaccurately or inappropriately. He or she may become sleepy, seem to doze off, and then suddenly wake up or become completely unconscious. Breathing may become fast and shallow or irregular, or may stop altogether because of paralysis in the nerves or muscles of the chest. If this happens, perform rescue breathing.

4. Control any external bleeding. Use dressings, direct pressure, and bandages (see p. 37).
5. Maintain normal body temperature. The body's temperature-maintenance mechanisms may become impaired, leaving the victim more susceptible to shock.

The head is particularly vulnerable to injury because it does not have the padding of muscle and fat found on most of the rest of the body.

Any head injury caused by a fall or a blow to the head should be taken seriously, since it could result in brain or spinal cord damage. Blood vessels inside the brain can be ruptured, causing pressure from the accumulation of blood, which then damages brain cells. Any victim found to be unconscious from unknown causes should be assumed to have a head injury—possible a neck injury as well—until his or her condition is otherwise determined by trained medical personnel.

If the victim does not lose consciousness and does not seek medical attention, delayed signs and symptoms of brain damage should be watched for carefully for 48 hours. If any of these appear—unconsciousness, change in pulse, difficulty in breathing, convulsions, severe vomiting, eye pupils of unequal size, generally poor or unhealthy appearance—medical attention should be sought immediately.

Specific Instructions for Monitoring Potential Closed Head Injuries:

1. A responsible person should remain with the patient for the first 24 hours.
2. Awaken the patient every 2 hours for the first 8 hours of sleep. Ask the patient his or her name, where he or she is, and the date.
3. Limit the patient's activity for 24 to 48 hours.
4. Give no sedatives or pain medication other than Tylenol, unless prescribed by the patient's doctor.
5. The patient should go to a hospital emergency department immediately if there is:

   - Unusual drowsiness or difficulty in arousing the patient during the first night
   - Persistent vomiting
   - Blurred vision
   - Severe headache not relieved by Tylenol
   - Stiff neck
   - Bleeding or clear fluid dripping from the ears or nose
   - Weakness of any limb or limbs
   - Convulsions
   - Unequal dilation of pupils

Concussion

A concussion is a temporary impairment of brain function that can be caused by any strong force to the head that jolts the brain within the skull. It may result in a very brief loss of consciousness, the sensation of "blacking out" or "seeing stars," confusion, amnesia, dizziness, or weakness. It usually does not cause permanent physical damage to brain tissue. Anyone suspected of having a concussion should be examined by a physician. Rest is usually suggested until the signs and symptoms disappear.

Skull Fracture

The skull may be fractured at any place on the head without any visible wound to the scalp. Such an injury is always considered serious because of the danger of possible brain damage. The victim of a skull fracture may exhibit any or all of the general signs and symptoms for head and spinal injuries, in addition to impaired vision or sudden blindness.

Treatment for a Skull Fracture:

1. Stabilize the head with your hands as you open the airway using the modified jaw-thrust maneuver (see p. 160).
2. Check breathing and give rescue breaths if necessary (see p. 161).
3. Check pulse.
4. If there is bleeding from the scalp, control it with direct pressure (see p. 37) and dress the wound; tie knots around the bandage away from the injured area. Do not try to control bleeding from the ears. Control bleeding from the nose only if no clear liquid (cerebrospinal fluid) is mixed with it.

5. Keep the victim quiet and lying down.
6. Immobilize the head and neck with your hands or with a rolled blanket or padding fastened around the head and neck.
7. Pad around the fractured area and under the neck to keep the victim's head from resting on the suspected fracture.
8. Maintain body temperature and treat for shock (see p. 305).

Neck Injuries

If there is an injury to the head, there is often an injury to the neck as well. *Never* move a victim with a suspected neck injury. Any movement of the head—back, forward, or side to side—can result in paralysis or death. A soft-tissue injury of the neck may cause severe bleeding and swelling that can block the airway. If the neck has been injured by running into a clothesline, the trachea may be fractured, obstructing the airway in a way that requires immediate medical attention.

Injuries of the Spine

Injuries of the head and neck very often involve injuries of the spine as well. Traumatic injury to a region of the spine can injure a set of nerves and paralyze a specific body area. Spinal injuries include fractures and dislocations of the vertebrae, sprained ligaments, and compressed or displaced disks. Vertebral fractures and ligament sprains usually heal without problems. If the force of an injury causes the vertebrae to shift and compress or severs the spinal cord, however, temporary or permanent paralysis, or even death, may result.

Because of this potential for morbidity and mortality, it is extremely important to be able to recognize the signs and symptoms of spinal column injuries. In addition to the general signs and symptoms of head and spinal injuries listed above, the following particularly relate to injuries of the spine.

Signs and Symptoms of Spine Injury:

➤ Pain and tenderness at the site of the injury
➤ Pain, tingling, or numbness at any point on the back, neck, or down the arms or legs
➤ Deformity
➤ Cuts and bruises
➤ Paralysis. If the victim is conscious, check for paralysis first in the lower extremities:

1. Ask the victim if he or she can feel your touch on his or her feet.
2. Ask the victim to wiggle his or her toes.
3. Ask the victim to press against your hands with his or her feet.

Then, check for paralysis in the upper extremities:

1. Ask the victim if he or she can feel your touch on his or her hands.
2. Ask the victim to wiggle his or her fingers.
3. Ask the victim to grasp your hand and squeeze.

If the victim is unconscious, test for paralysis as follows:

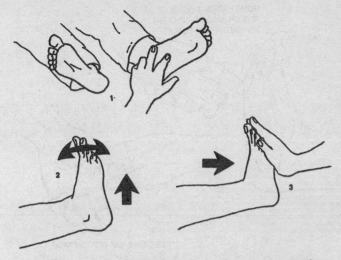

Checking for Paralysis in the Lower Extremities When the Victim is Conscious

1. Stroke the soles of the feet or the ankles with a pointed object. If the spinal cord is undamaged, the feet will react.
2. Stroke the palms of the hand with a pointed object. If the spinal cord is undamaged, the hands will react.

Treat a spinal injury by following the general rules for head, neck, and spine injuries (see p. 209). The most important things to remember are to immobilize the injured area, to keep the victim as still as possible, to maintain an open airway, and to control bleeding.

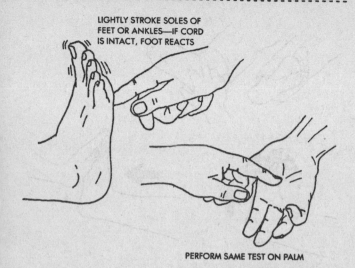

LIGHTLY STROKE SOLES OF
FEET OR ANKLES—IF CORD
IS INTACT, FOOT REACTS

PERFORM SAME TEST ON PALM

Checking for Paralysis (Unconscious Victim)

Tips for Preventing Head, Neck, and Spine Injuries:

- Wear safety belts when riding in an automobile, and put children in approved safety seats.
- Wear appropriate protective helmets when riding a motorcycle or bicycle.
- Wear protective eye wear when using machinery or performing an activity that may involve flying particles or splashing chemicals.
- Periodically inspect mechanical equipment and ladders to make certain they are in good working order, checking for worn, broken, or loose parts that could give way and cause an accident. Before climbing a ladder, place its legs

on a firm, flat surface and have someone hold it while you climb.

- Follow the tips for preventing falls under Tips for Preventing Dislocations and Fractures, p. 151.

Heart Attack and Cardiac Arrest

The heart is a fist-sized muscular organ that works like a pump, sending oxygen-rich blood to all the cells in the body and receiving oxygen-depleted blood back, which it then sends to the lungs to be reoxygenated. The reoxygenated blood comes back into the heart from the lungs and is then pumped out again. The coronary arteries supply the cells of the heart itself with oxygenated blood. When this supply is reduced, cells of the heart muscle start to die. When so much heart tissue dies that the heart cannot pump effectively, the condition is known as a heart attack. Cardiac arrest occurs when the heart stops beating or beats too irregularly or too weakly to circulate blood effectively throughout the body.

Cardiovascular disease—disease of the heart and blood vessels—is the most frequent cause of heart attacks and cardiac arrest. The most common form of this disease is atherosclerosis, which occurs when fatty deposits build up on the interior wall of the arteries, particularly the coronary arteries, which nourish the cells of the heart. Diet and exercise have been shown to be major factors in preventing atherosclerosis.

Of the more than 540,000 people in the United States who die every year of heart attacks, approximately 350,000 die outside the hospital within the first 2 hours after cardiac arrest. This makes recognition of heart attack signs and symptoms extremely important in preventing heart-attack mortality.

Note: Signs and symptoms of a heart attack, though they may follow the classic pattern outlined below, also frequently present with very atypical symptoms. Any patient experiencing chest pain should seek medical attention.

Classic Signs and Symptoms of a Heart Attack:

➤ Persistent central chest pain or discomfort. The pain is usually crushing (not stabbing) and may last for several minutes. It may be confused with chest pain caused by indigestion, muscle spasms, or other conditions. If the pain is brief and sharp or intensifies when the victim bends over or inhales deeply, it is probably not caused by a heart attack.

The discomfort may manifest as pressure, tightness, aching, or heaviness. The sensation in the chest may spread to the shoulder, arm, neck, jaw, midback, or pit of the stomach and is usually not relieved by resting or changing position. Any chest pain or severe discomfort that lasts for more than 10 minutes or is accompanied by any other heart attack signs and symptoms should receive immediate emergency medical care.

➤ Shortness of breath or very fast breathing. The victim may begin breathing faster and gasping for air in an attempt to get more oxygen into his or her system.

➤ Sweating, particularly on the face
➤ Pale or bluish cast to the skin, especially of the face
➤ Irregular pulse, or pulse rate that is faster or slower than usual. A heart attack interrupts the heart's electrical system, which controls the pulse.
➤ Nausea
➤ Feeling of weakness

Heart-attack victims may deny the seriousness of their condition, so your observation of the signs and symptoms and insistence upon taking immediate action is critical in preventing further damage or death.

Treatment for a Heart Attack If Victim Is Conscious (Cardiac Arrest Has Not Occurred):

1. Call EMS personnel. Survival may depend upon how quickly advanced medical care is received. Do *not* try to drive the victim to the hospital yourself, since cardiac arrest could occur en route and you would be unable to observe and treat it.
2. Have the victim stop whatever activity he or she is engaged in and gently place him or her in a comfortable position—sitting up or in a semi-reclining posture, using pillows, if available, for greater comfort. Do *not* have the victim lie down flat, because this may make it more difficult for him or her to breathe.
3. Loosen tight clothing, especially around the victim's neck and abdomen.

4. Cover the victim with a blanket or overcoat to keep him or her comfortably warm.
5. Calm and reassure the victim.
6. Do *not* give the victim anything to eat or drink.

Signs and Symptoms of Cardiac Arrest:

➤ No discernible breathing
➤ Absence of pulse

Seattle, Washington, has a cardiac arrest survival rate that is more than five times the national average. It is probably no coincidence that all Seattle firefighters are also trained as EMTs and that a very high percentage of the population has taken CPR courses. On the night of May 5, 1993, Jim Knox, a 55-year-old air traffic controller at Sea-Tac International Airport outside Seattle, had particular cause to be very grateful for this.

Jim sat in a darkened room with two other controllers, watching lights move across his radar screen. Ed Gass, air traffic controller supervisor on duty that night, described the scene. "Aircraft are coming in toward the radar controllers from all points of the compass," said Gass. "Their job is to position the aircraft so that, ultimately, the airplanes end up one behind the other in an orderly fashion and land one at a time. They depend on us to provide safe instructions. There's a lot of stress associated with the job." Jim had responsibility for all aircraft approaching from the west.

Dick Bobb, the traffic manager on duty and one of Jim's oldest friends, noticed—as he made his tour of the room, checking with the controllers to see if anyone needed help—that Jim was slumped forward with his head resting on his control board. Just a short while before, he had stopped at Jim's console to tease him amiably about his impending retirement. "Jim's like a brother to me," he said. "We've known each other a long time—18 years. Our kids grew up together—we're damn good friends!"

"Traffic that slow, Jimmy?" Dick quipped, hoping that his friend was just playing a practical joke, pretending to be asleep. To his alarm, Jim did not respond. "Jimmy, can you hear me?" he shouted. Still, there was no response.

Sue Hoover, one of the other controllers on duty, recognized the gravity of the situation, but could not immediately leave her console to help. "Jimmy was definitely in distress, but you couldn't stop what you were doing—there were too many people up there," she said, referring to the planes and pilots depending on her for direction and instruction.

Supervisor Ed Gass came over to Jim, lifted his head, and realized that he was unconscious. Gass instructed Mike Callahan, the third controller on duty, to pull in Jim's radar frequency to his equipment and take over the planes Jim should have been handling. He told Dick Bobb, "Call 9-1-1. I think Jimmy's had a heart attack," and carefully laid Jim on the floor, face up, on his back.

"Does anybody know CPR?" another controller who had come into the room asked.

"I do," Sue Hoover responded, "but it's been a while." The other controller took over for Sue, who went to join Ed to administer two-person CPR to their stricken and unconscious colleague. Ed checked Jim for a pulse, but wasn't able to find one.

"I was nervous because I wasn't sure if I remembered the numbers right—how many breaths and how many compressions," Sue said. "So I gave him a couple of breaths and then checked for a pulse. I didn't find one and then it really sank in, just what was going on—his heart was stopped." Sue then did chest compressions, trading off with Ed when she got tired.

"I was concerned because Jimmy's life was literally in the hands of a couple of amateurs," Ed said. "We hoped we were doing the right thing, but we had no assurance that we were."

"I would just as soon somebody else had done it, but I was the best chance he had at that point," Sue said, "so I tried. But I was really worried that what I was doing was hurting him more than helping him." In spite of her anxiety, Sue kept working on her lifeless colleague. "Come on, Jimmy, come on," she urged.

Within minutes of Dick Bobb's 9-1-1 call, a Sea-Tac Airport rescue team of EMTs arrived in the control room, and took over the task of performing CPR from Ed and Sue, working in the semidarkness so that the controllers could continue to read their radar screens. The challenge, quite simply, was to save Jim's life without endangering those of the thousands of people waiting in the air to land. In the cramped space on the floor of the room, the EMTs decided to defibrillate Jim—a process in which an electrical shock is sent to the heart to enable it to resume a functional heartbeat.

"I was hoping that they'd defibrillate Jim and they'd have a heartbeat," Sue said. "But it didn't work. They did it once, and then they did it again. At that point, I couldn't watch anymore."

Approximately 10 minutes after Jim's heart attack, a county life-support team of paramedics arrived. "The people that I met as I entered the room asked me if we could move the patient," said the team leader, a little incredulously. "I told them that right now he was straddling the fence between life and death, and until he puts his foot down on one side or the other, we're going to have to work on him right here." The paramedics gave Jim a drug intravenously to keep him from refibrillating (returning to a chaotic, fluttering heartbeat, after which the heart stops altogether), and defibrillated him two more times. On the second try, they were successful in getting his heart to pick up a rhythmic beat that would sustain a pulse and keep up his blood pressure on its own. From the control room, Jim was transported to Highline Community Hospital.

"The scariest thing was watching them roll him out of there, and wondering if I'd ever see him again," said Dick Bobb, "wondering if I'd ever again have the Jimmy that I knew." Dick followed the ambulance to the hospital, where he was joined by Jim's wife, Jane. "She asked me how he was, and I told her that he was in the emergency room, unconscious, and that the doctors said he'd had a heart attack. She broke down. I gave her a hug and we cried together," Dick said.

"You're going to be all right. It will be all right," Jane soothingly told her unconscious husband.

"I was terrified. Here was a man who was the strength of the family, whom we all look up to. It was just terrifying to see him down like that. If I'd lost him, I would have been . . ." Jane said, letting her voice trail off, unable to finish the sentence.

Curtis Burnett, the cardiologist who took over Jim's care, acknowledged the importance of the work Ed Gass, Sue Hoover, the EMTs, and the paramedics had done. "In this case, we're basically in a supporting function," he said. "The work to save Jim's life happened out in the field, and we're here to do what we can to prevent [the problem] from recurring."

Finally, someone came to tell Dick, Jane, and Ed, who had joined them at the hospital, that Jim was awake and talking.

Jim ultimately had a device implanted that automatically delivers an electrical shock to his heart anytime it stops beating, and went onto enjoy his much-anticipated retirement. "I feel great," he said 5 months after the heart attack. "I don't feel any different now from before it happened."

"We're very fortunate," Jane said. "The doctor told us that if he had not had the immediate CPR, he would have been either dead or brain damaged, period. We've become almost inseparable. We simply just enjoy each other's company—and he's my life."

If a victim is not breathing and has no pulse, he or she is in cardiac arrest, also known as "sudden death." Although heart attacks are the most common cause of cardiac arrest, it can also be brought on by severe injury to the chest, extreme loss of blood, electrocution, drowning, stroke, or other forms of brain damage. The key symptom is the absence of a pulse.

Although a person in cardiac arrest is "clinically dead," vital organs can continue to live for a short period of time using the oxygen stored in the blood-stream. Cardiopulmonary resuscitation, or CPR (*Cardio-*, "of the heart," plus *pulmonary,* "of the lungs"), is a way of artificially taking over the functions of circulation and breathing, so that air continues to come into the body and blood continues to flow. Without this assistance, brain-cell death will begin within 4 to 6 minutes, usually causing irreversible brain damage.

CPR alone will not save a cardiac-arrest victim, since it can supply only one-third of the normal supply of blood to the brain, but it is *essential* to maintaining life until advanced medical care is available.

Caution: CPR, the primary first-aid treatment for cardiac emergencies, should be studied and practiced under professional supervision. Courses are available through the American Heart Association and the American Red Cross. Incorrect application of the procedure could result in damage to internal organs, bone fractures, or separation of cartilage from bone. If performed when not required, it can result in cardiac arrest, so *never* practice CPR on another person. (Dummies are used in the courses.)

CPR for an Adult:

1. Call EMS personnel for help.
2. Assess the situation to establish unresponsive-

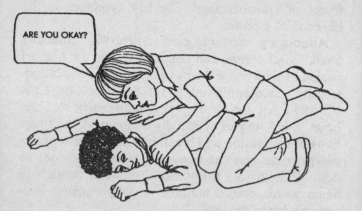

Recognition of the Problem

ness by gently shaking the victim's shoulder and shouting, "Are you okay?"

3. If the victim is not lying on his or her back, position the victim so that he or she is, on a firm, flat surface. If there is any indication of head or spinal injury, maintain spinal alignment and immobilize the victim (see pp. 209–10).

4. **A—Airway.** Open the airway with the head-tilt/chin-lift maneuver, unless you suspect a head or spinal injury (see p. 160).

5. **B—Breathing.** Establish that the victim is not breathing and give two slow rescue breaths—1½ to 2 seconds each (see p. 161).

6. **C—Circulation.** Check for a pulse. Kneeling at the victim's side, with one hand tilting his or her forehead back to maintain an open airway, put two fingertips of your other hand on the

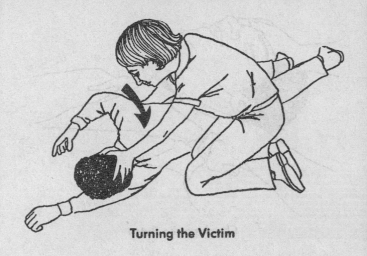

Turning the Victim

victim's windpipe, then slowly slide them back toward you until you reach the groove of the neck. Press gently on this area (carotid artery). Check the pulse here for at least 5 seconds, but no more than 10. If there is no pulse:

7. Perform cardiac compressions.

   a. Kneel beside the victim's chest, making certain that his or her head is on the same level as his or her heart or lower so that blood flow to the brain will not be reduced.

   b. Locate the bottom of the victim's rib cage with the index and middle fingers of one hand. Run these fingers up along the edge of the rib cage to the notch where the ribs meet the breastbone. Place your index finger on the sternum and the middle finger next to it in the notch.

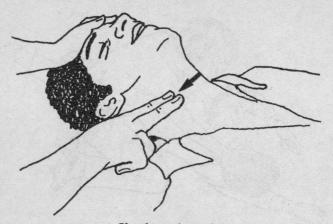

Checking the Pulse

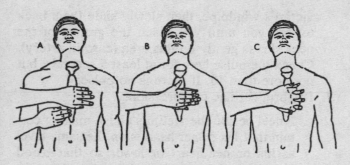

Correct Hand Position on the Sternum

c. Put the heel of the other hand on the breastbone just above your index finger, in the center of the sternum, with the fingers pointing
away from you.

d. Place the hand you used to locate the notch

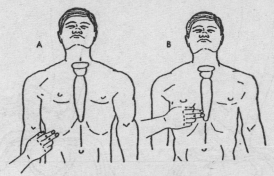

Locating the Xiphoid Process

directly on top of the hand on the sternum and parallel to it. Interlock fingers or tilt them upward to keep them off the chest. If you have arthritis or a similar condition, you may also grasp the wrist of the hand positioned on the chest with your other hand.

Caution: The correct hand position is extremely important. There is an arrow-shaped piece of hard tissue at the bottom of the sternum called the xiphoid. You should avoid putting pressure directly on the xiphoid, which can break and cause damage to underlying tissue.

e. Lean forward and position your shoulders directly over your hands, locking your elbows, so that pressure will be exerted directly downward.

f. Compress the chest about 1½ to 2 inches, using the weight of your upper body to push the heel of your hand downward. This will squeeze the heart between the spine and the

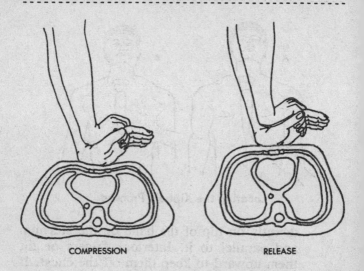

COMPRESSION   RELEASE

Cardiac Compressions

sternum, emptying the chambers of the heart and pumping blood through the body.

g. Release the pressure completely, maintaining contact between the heel of your hand and the victim's chest, to allow the heart to refill with blood.

The compression and release should be done in a smooth manner, without rocking back and forth. Perform 15 compressions and releases, counting "1 and 2 and . . ." up to 15. (The rate is about 80 to 100 compressions per minute.) If you find yourself tiring, you may not be in the correct position, or may be using pressure from your muscles instead of the weight of your upper body. Otherwise, little effort should be required.

8. Do the head-tilt/chin-lift to open the airway, and give two slow rescue breaths (see p. 161).

9. Repeat the cycle of compressions and rescue breathing three more times so that you have done four cycles in all.

10. After the fourth cycle of 15 compressions and 2 breaths, tilt the victim's head back to open the airway and check the carotid artery for a pulse (3 to 5 seconds). This will tell you if the heart has started beating.

11. If pulse is absent, continue the compression-and-breathing cycle, stopping every few minutes to check again for the pulse. Do *not* stop CPR for more than 5 seconds for any other reason, until qualified medical personnel arrive.

If you find a pulse, check for breathing and give rescue breaths if needed. Continue to monitor for heartbeat and breathing until EMS personnel arrive.

If the victim starts to vomit during CPR, roll the victim on his or her side, turning the whole body as a unit. Clear out the mouth with your fingers. Roll the victim back onto his or her back, tilt his or her head backward to open the airway, give two rescue breaths, and resume CPR cycles of compression and breathing.

CPR for a Child (1 to 8 Years of Age):

CPR for a child is similar to that for an adult with two important exceptions:

1. Only one hand is used for the compressions. The other is kept on the victim's forehead.
2. One rescue breath is given after every five compressions.

CPR for an Infant:

1. Establish unresponsiveness by the shake and shout method.
2. Check for any foreign matter in the mouth and remove it.
3. Open the airway, being careful not to over-extend the neck.
4. Cover the infant's nose and mouth with your lips to get an airtight seal.
5. Puff cheeks, using the air in your mouth to give two quick rescue breaths.
6. Check the brachial pulse. Keeping the palm of one hand on the infant's forehead so that the head is tilted slightly backward and the airway is kept open, place the tips of the index and middle fingers of your other hand on the inner side of the upper arm. Press lightly on the arm at the groove in the muscle. If there is no pulse, start CPR immediately, by taking the following steps.
7. Place the infant on his or her back on a firm, level surface with his or her head on the same level as his or her body or slightly lower.
8. Place the palm of one of your hands on the infant's forehead, tilting the head very slightly back to keep the airway open.
9. Place two of your three middle fingers about a

finger width below the midpoint of an imaginary line joining the infant's nipples.

10. Keeping the other hand on the infant's forehead, perform five compressions by pushing down on the infant's chest with your fingers to a depth of ½ to 1 inch and releasing, letting the chest rise without removing your fingers. The rate should be somewhat faster than for an adult (*at least* 100 compressions per minute) because an infant's heart beats faster. Set the rhythm by counting 1 and 2 and . . ." out loud.

11. Give one rescue breath as described above (steps 4 and 5).

12. Repeat the cycle of compressions and breathing 19 more times.

13. Activate the EMS system (you will now have done 20 cycles in all).

14. Check for a pulse.

15. If there is no pulse, continue CPR with the five compressions, one breath cycle until the infant starts to breathe and his or her heart starts to beat, or until EMS personnel arrive. If there is a pulse but no breathing, give rescue breaths at the rate of one breath every 3 seconds.

If vomiting occurs, turn the infant on his or her side, clean out his or her mouth with your fingers, return the infant to his or her back, and tilt the head backward slightly to open the airway. Resume rescue breathing and chest compressions if necessary.

Do not stop CPR for more than 5 seconds except to check for a pulse or clear the airway after vomiting.

PR with Two Trained Rescuers:

1. If one rescuer is tired, the second may take over by kneeling next to the victim on the opposite side from the first.
2. When the first rescuer completes a cycle of compressions and breaths, the second rescuer tilts the head of the victim with one hand and checks the carotid pulse.
3. If there is no pulse, the second rescuer takes over performing the CPR cycles.
4. The first rescuer watches the chest during rescue breathing to make certain it is rising and falling and checks the carotid pulse for an artificial beat during the compressions to make certain that blood is being moved through the victim's body.

Heat Emergencies

Heat cramps, heat exhaustion, and heatstroke are conditions of increasing severity resulting from overexposure to heat. Heat cramps, the least severe, can lead to heat exhaustion and heatstroke.

Treatment for Heat Emergencies:

1. Cool the body.
2. Give fluids.
3. Minimize shock.

Heat cramps are pains and spasms in skeletal muscles, probably brought on by a loss of salt and fluid in the body due to heavy sweating. They generally affect people who perform strenuous physical activity in a hot environment and perspire heavily, and tend to develop rapidly, often immediately after the exertion. They can also occur in warm or even moderate temperatures if the activity is intense and sustained. The muscles of the stomach and the legs are usually affected first, but the cramps can occur in any voluntary muscle. Heat cramps may also be symptomatic of heat exhaustion or heat stroke.

Signs and Symptoms of Heat Cramps:

➤ Muscle cramps and/or severe convulsions in the legs and/or abdomen
➤ Profuse sweating
➤ Possible faintness
➤ Possible convulsions
➤ Normal body temperature (unless cramps are symptomatic of more severe heat injury)

Treatment for Heat Cramps:

1. Move the victim to a cool environment and have him or her sit there quietly.
2. Apply firm hand pressure to the affected areas or gently massage the victim's cramped muscles.
3. If the victim is conscious and not vomiting, give him or her sips of clear juice or cool salt and sugar water (1 teaspoon of salt plus as much sugar as the person can stand) or a commercial electrolyte solution. If these are not available, give plain cool water. Give half a glass of liquid every 15 minutes for 1 hour, unless the victim starts vomiting.
4. If the victim starts vomiting, place him or her on his or her side.

Heat exhaustion can occur after long exposure to high temperatures, particularly if accompanied by high humidity, which results in the excessive loss of water and salt. It is usually associated with athletes, but can also affect firefighters, construction workers, factory workers, and others who wear hot, heavy clothing in a hot, humid environment. It also commonly occurs in people not accustomed to hot weather, people who are overweight, and people who perspire excessively. It is an early indication that environmental conditions are overwhelming the body's ability to regulate temperature. The effect on the circulatory system causes the victim to go into mild shock.

Signs and Symptoms of Heat Exhaustion:

➤ Cool, clammy, pale (slightly blanched if the victim is very dark skinned), or red skin
➤ Profuse perspiration
➤ Elevated or below-normal body temperature
➤ Rapid, shallow breathing
➤ Possible headache, nausea, dizziness, and/or weakness
➤ Rapid and weak pulse
➤ Exhaustion
➤ Possible muscle cramps
➤ Possible vomiting
➤ Possible fainting

Treatment for Heat Exhaustion:

1. Move the victim to a cool and comfortable place, or at the very least into the shade, but do not allow chilling.
2. Try to cool the victim immediately by fanning

and/or wiping his or her face with a cool, wet cloth.

3. Loosen any tight clothing and remove clothing soaked with sweat.

4. Place cool, wet cloths (such as towels or sheets if available) on the victim's skin, and fan the victim to increase evaporation.

5. If the victim is not vomiting, give clear juice or sips of cool salt water (1 teaspoon of salt per glass), half glass every 15 minutes for 1 hour. If these are not available, give plain water. Stop if the victim starts to vomit, and place him or her on his or her side.

6. If fainting seems likely, have the victim lie down, with his or her feet elevated 8 to 12 inches.

7. Treat the victim for shock (see p. 305).

8. If signs and symptoms are severe, become worse, or last for more than 1 hour, seek medical attention.

9. Do not allow the victim to resume normal activities the same day.

Heatstroke (also known as sunstroke) can come on quite suddenly and most often occurs when people ignore the signs of heat exhaustion. It is a life-threatening emergency that develops when the body's temperature-regulating mechanisms are overwhelmed by heat from direct exposure to the rays of the sun or extremely high temperatures without exposure to the sun. Humidity and physical exertion contribute substantially to the incidence of heatstroke. The body's fluids become so depleted that perspiration stops and the body can no longer cool itself effectively, resulting in a rapid rise of body temperature. It soon reaches a level at which the brain and other vital organs begin to fail. If the body is not cooled and these effects are not reversed, convulsions, coma, and death will result. The condition is more common among the elderly, the obese, alcoholics, and those on medication.

Given extreme environmental conditions, anyone can become vulnerable to heatstroke, as Sandi Taylor of Las Vegas, Nevada, learned one afternoon on what her boyfriend had planned as a romantic outing.

On the morning of July 7, 1990, 28-year-old David Jones and Sandi, his 19-year-old girlfriend, headed out for the Red Rock Canyon National Conservation Area, less than 10 miles from Las Vegas. They had been going out together for only a few months, and on that day David planned to take Sandi hiking along one of his favorite trails. "Red Rock Canyon is an absolutely beautiful place to be," David said. "Because it's very isolated, it tends to be romantic, so it was a good opportunity for us to get to know each other a little bit better." When they got to the point where they were to leave their car and start the hike, David checked the supplies while Sandi debated whether she should wear a hat her father had given her to keep the sun off her head. "But she really didn't like how it looked," David said. So in spite of the bright sun and the intense heat (which would reach well over 105° Fahrenheit that day), Sandi decided not to wear it.

"The going was pretty easy at first," David said. "But progressively, it got more and more difficult. It was hot. The temperature was easily over 100 degrees. Sandi is a less experienced hiker than I am, but she just kept going."

When they stopped to eat their sandwiches, Sandi realized the effort of the hike had left her famished. "I am so hungry that anything would taste good," she told David. After lunch, they decided to hike back down the canyon.

"Are you okay, Sandi?" David asked as they started out again. "Sandi?"

"Yeah, I'm okay," she responded, but with a note of fatigue in her voice.

"The sun was directly over our heads," David recalled, "so it was getting a little bit hotter."

After they'd walked for a while, David asked Sandi again if she was okay. "You know, I'm really tired," she said weakly. "Could we just sit down for a minute?"

David was resistant. "Sandi, if we stop, what are we going to do?" he asked.

"Both of us were now really hot. I didn't realize how bad the heat can be or what it can do to you. The water that we had was almost gone by this time. I felt it was better just to push it and get to the truck," he later explained.

"We're almost to the truck," he told Sandi. "Air conditioning as soon as we get there." Then, suddenly, Sandi, who had been walking behind, came hurtling past him down the trail. "Sandi, what are you doing?" David cried out in surprise.

"All of a sudden, she just took off, running down the trail," he said. Then she collapsed, and David rushed to her side. "When I got to her, she was incoherent and her face was very, very red. I had no idea what was going on with her," he said.

"Sandi, are you okay? Talk to me!" David said desperately. "Here, come on, let's get up. Come on!" he said. "We're almost to the car." But Sandi just lay there. "Come on! Come on!" David urged again, trying to drag her to her feet.

"We had not seen another person in our whole hike, the whole day. I didn't know whether I should leave her and go get some help. I didn't know which way to turn."

Providentially, 17-year-old Melissa Durfee and her boyfriend, Jim Thacker, also happened to be hiking the same trial, and within a few seconds they came around a bend and discovered David and Sandi. "Hey, you guys, come here, I need some help," David called out to them.

"When I saw her, something just clicked in my mind that it was from the heat," Melissa said. "We had almost turned back ourselves because it was just too much."

"She was complaining about how hot it was," David told them, trying to describe what had happened.

"When I touched her she was red and puffy," Jim said. "She was scary hot." The three of them lifted Sandi up and carried her to the shade of a small tree, which offered some protection from the sun.

"We knew we needed to get her temperature down, so we got her to some shade," Melissa said. "Then we started pouring water on her head. We just assumed that she would wake up—right away. But the longer it took, the more frightened we became." Sandi began throwing up, and the three of them began to sense the seriousness of the situation.

"She wasn't coming out of it. We decided this was pretty bad," said Jim. "We kept the water on her neck and on her chest area and over her head. Her skin ate the water up—it was that hot. We wrapped up her head so that it would hold the water to her, but she still wasn't coming out of it. I started to think that this person might not make it. There was a ranger station several miles down the road. We decided to go get help."

"You'll be okay. You'll be fine," David said to Sandi. "They'll be back in a few minutes. You'll be okay."

"I tried to talk to her," he said later, "and there was absolutely nothing—no response. I kept thinking, why didn't I just listen to her? I kept hearing her voice saying over and over, 'Why don't we just stop? Why don't we just rest for a while?' All of this could have been avoided, but I just kept pushing."

More than 30 minutes passed before the hikers returned with help, including Spring Mountain Ranch park ranger Jim Black. "It was almost immediately apparent that this woman was suffering from heatstroke," said Black, "which mans you're basically burning up inside. Her body was extremely overheated and had lost its ability to regulate its temperature. This is a condition where someone might die in just a very few minutes before your eyes."

Realizing that Sandi needed immediate medical attention, the rangers radioed for a Flight for Life helicopter, which arrived within 20 minutes. Flight nurse Chris Adams quickly took charge at the scene. "What's going on? What have we got?" she asked Black.

"Heatstroke," was the immediate reply.

"Her condition was very serious," said Adams, "considering that they'd been cooling her aggressively for at least half an hour. Her temperature was very high—104.5. You literally are just kind of cooking the tissues in your different organs." She gave Sandi oxygen and fluids intravenously to rehydrate her and placed iced packs at critical points on her body, as Sandi struggled against the tube they were putting down her throat. "I needed to cool her down as quickly a possible. I applied ice packs and I started the IV line to help rehydrate her, but I've never seen a heatstroke victim that's lost consciousness survive—particularly one with as high a temperature as she had."

"Sandi, even though she was unconscious, she was fighting," David said. "And I knew at that point in time, even though we'd just been dating for a very short period, that this girl had a tremendous strength inside."

Sandi was loaded onto the helicopter and transported to Valley Hospital Medical Center, where she arrived in a coma with a body temperature of 105° Fahrenheit; and was placed under the care of emergency physician Tony Frederick. "We immediately applied cool compresses over her entire body," Frederick said, "and had fans blowing on her because evaporation is the most efficient means to cool these patients. However, her condition did not really improve. I felt that this woman could easily die or have permanent brain damage." Sandi was kept in the intensive care unit, where doctors continued to monitor the swelling of her brain.

Sandi's parents, Bob and Suzanne Taylor, came to the hospital as soon as they were notified. "When I saw her, my heart just sank," said Sandi's mother. "You would talk to her, and her eyes were wide open, but there was nothing there."

"All of your hopes and dreams are wrapped in your first child," Sandi's father said. "All the things that you ever wanted for her, you see the possibility of that being snuffed out. I could never imagine not having her there with us."

"We're all deeply religious," David said, "and so the first thing that we thought of was to give her a blessing. We had to put our faith in God to help Sandi pull through this. And the next morning, her mother greeted me and said, 'David, she's out of the coma, and it looks like she's going to be okay.'"

Miraculously, Sandi beat the odds and made a complete recovery, with no sign of brain damage. Six months after the incident, she and David were married.

"When you're in a situation where someone's life is in danger, there is a strong bond that is created," David said. "Sandi is just a beautiful person. She's fun to be around. She really is a great companion to me. The friendship that we've had and the love that we've shared with each other has been absolutely incredible. My life today is so much richer and so much fuller."

"I just remember that it was really hot," Sandi said. "I felt like my head was frying, but I didn't know that 'Gee, this is a sign of heatstroke, so I'd better really be careful.' I should have slowed down and I should have drunk a lot more, but I didn't want to be embarrassed by the fact that I was feeling kind of sick. I never blamed David for what happened."

"Sandi is one of the very few and very lucky people who recover 100% fully from this type of heatstroke," Bob Taylor, Sandi's father, said. "If you're going to go out and be exposed to these kinds of temperatures, have plenty of water, and you have to take protection from the sun. Wear a hat—and most important of all, listen to your father."

"I look at my baby daughter Sarah sometimes and think that if David hadn't been there for me or if those hikers hadn't been there—if one person had been missing in the whole rescue, then she wouldn't be here at all," Sandi said. "I never would have gotten off that mountain without any of those people. And so I'm very grateful to all of them because I owe everything I have to them."

Signs and Symptoms of Heatstroke:

➤ Very high body temperature (often 106° Fahrenheit or higher)
➤ Red, hot, and very dry skin. In the case of very dark skinned people, the change in skin color is not as perceptible. Perspiration is usually absent.
➤ Strong, rapid pulse, which can become weak and rapid if the victim's condition worsens. The heart first works hard to rid the body of heat by dilating blood vessels and sending more blood to the skin. As consciousness begins to fail, so does the circulatory system and the pulse becomes weak.
➤ Rapid, deep breathing followed by rapid, shallow breathing
➤ Progressive loss of consciousness or increasing confusion
➤ Possible convulsions

Treatment for Heatstroke:

1. Call EMS personnel.
2. Maintain an open airway (see p. 160).

3. Remove the victim to a cool environment.
4. Remove all the victim's clothing.
5. Cool the victim by any means available. If the victim is conscious and can be monitored, put him or her in a tub of cold (not iced) water. If the victim is unconscious or consciousness is decreasing, soak towels or sheets and apply them to the victim's body instead, so that it will be possible to maintain an open airway. If ice packs or cold packs are available, place them on each wrist and ankle, on the groin, in each armpit, and on the neck to cool the large blood vessels. If this is not possible, you can also spray the skin with a hose or sponge it with cool water. Do *not* apply rubbing alcohol, which closes the skin's pores and prevents heat loss.
6. Continue treatment until body temperature is 101° or 102° Farenheit. Do *not* overchill. Check body temperature constantly.
7. Dry off the victim once his or her temperature is lowered.
8. Place the victim in front of a fan or air conditioner to continue cooling.
9. If the body temperature rises again, repeat the cooling process.
10. Do *not* give the victim alcoholic beverages or stimulants such as coffee or tea.

If a person is suffering from heat cramps or heat exhaustion and refuses water, starts to vomit, or starts to lose consciousness, these are clear signs that his or her condition is worsening, and EMS personnel should be called immediately.

Tips for Preventing Heat Emergencies:

- Avoid being outdoors at the hottest part of the day.
- Avoid doing heavy exercise at the hottest part of the day.
- Alter your activity level according to the outdoor temperature, wind, and rain.
- Take frequent breaks to allow the body to readjust its temperature-maintenance mechanisms.
- Dress appropriately for the environment.
- Drink large amounts of fluids.
- Do *not* drink alcohol or take any drug or medication that might lower your awareness of temperature extremes if you are planning to be outdoors in extremely hot or humid weather.

Hyperventilation

Hyperventilation occurs when someone breathes faster and more deeply than normal. This disturbs the body's balance of oxygen and carbon dioxide, lowering the level of carbon dioxide in the blood. This may cause muscle tightness in the throat and chest, which often increases the panic that the victim is already experiencing. Hyperventilation is frequently brought on by fear or anxiety and is more common in people who are tense or nervous. Other common triggers are injuries (such as head injuries), severe bleeding, illnesses (such as high fever, heart failure, lung disease, diabetes, and asthma), and exercise.

Signs and Symptoms of Hyperventilation:

➤ A sense by the victim that he or she cannot get enough air and is suffocating
➤ Lightheadedness
➤ Dizziness
➤ Numbness and tingling in fingers and toes and around the mouth and lips

➤ Possible muscle twitching
➤ Possible convulsions

Treatment for Hyperventilation:

1. If you suspect the cause is emotional, calm and reassure the victim.
2. Place a brown paper bag loosely over the victim's nose and throat so that he or she can breathe the air and carbon monoxide mixture, causing the muscles to relax. Have him or her continue to do this for 4 or 5 minutes, exhaling slowly. Alternatively, have the victim cup both hands around his or her mouth and nose and breathe into them.
3. If breathing does not return to normal or if the victim becomes unconscious, call EMS personnel immediately. A pulmonary embolism, which is a life-threatening condition requiring immediate medical attention, may be present.

Mouth and Teeth Injuries

An injury to the mouth can cause breathing problems if blood or loose teeth obstruct the airway. If there are no signs and symptoms of a serious head or spinal injury, have the victim sit down with his or her head tilted forward slightly to allow blood to drain. If this is painful or uncomfortable, have the victim lie on his or her side to facilitate drainage.

If an injury has penetrated the lip, place a rolled dressing between the lip and the gums, and another dressing on the outer surface of the lip. If the tongue is bleeding, apply a dressing and direct pressure. Apply cold to the lips or tongue to reduce swelling and pain.

Treatment for Knocked-Out Teeth:

If the tooth cannot be found, is destroyed, or is a baby tooth:

1. Control bleeding by rolling a sterile dressing and inserting it into the space left by the missing tooth. Have the victim bite down to maintain pressure.

2. Wrap the tooth in a cool, wet cloth. Do *not* place it in tap water, which has minerals that may further damage the tooth. A saline solution (salt dissolved in water) may be used.

3. Transport the victim and the tooth to a dentist or hospital emergency room as quickly as possible. Time is critical for a successful replantation. Ideally, the tooth should be replanted within an hour of the injury.

If the tooth is an adult tooth and is undamaged, place it back in the tooth socket and, pressing it firmly in place, seek immediate dental help. If the tooth has fallen on the ground, rinse it with cool water to remove any dirt before placing it back into the tooth socket.

Poisoning

A poison is any substance that produces a harmful effect on the body when it enters it. A poison can cause injury, illness, or death, depending upon how strong it is, the amount of it introduced into the victim's system, the length of time it stays in the system, and the victim's physical condition. The measure of the strength of a poison is called toxicity. Poisons include solids, liquids, and fumes, and can enter the body in four ways:

- Ingestion (eating or drinking)
- Inhalation (breathing through the nose or the mouth)
- Injection (into the body tissues or the bloodstream) (see Bites and Stings, p. 9)
- Absorption (through the skin)

Every year more than 4,000 people in America die from poisoning. It is such a unique and widespread health problem that the Poison Control Centers network has been created around the country. These centers are staffed by medical professionals who have access to information about virtually all poisonous substances and can tell you how to counteract a poison. You can obtain the phone number of your local Poison Control Center from the telephone directory, your doctor, a local hospital, or your local EMS system. This number should be posted by your phone. If it is not, and you have a poisoning emergency to deal with, call your local emergency number and ask to be connected with the local Poison Control Center.

POISONING BY INGESTION

Ingested poisons include foods, such as certain mushrooms or shellfish; improperly stored foods; medications taken inappropriately, in too-large doses, or mixed with alcohol; alcohol itself; and household and garden items, such as cleaning products, pesticides, and plants. The major causes of poisoning by ingestion are:

- Overdose of medication, intentional or accidental, including combining drugs with alcohol when this is contraindicated
- Household cleaners, chemicals, and medications left within the reach of children
- Original labels left on containers now used to store poisons
- Improperly stored food

 In December 1984, Sarah Bedore and her family in Windham, Connecticut, discovered the dangers of leaving a child alone, however briefly, when medicine is left in an easily accessible place.

"I was babysitting for my granddaughter, Sharelle, while her mother was in the hospital having another baby," Sarah said, recounted the event. "I thought that this was going to be great, because I would be able to have a whole lot of time with her." Sarah shared the house where 2-year-old Sharelle was visiting her with the child's 84-year-old great-grandmother, who was nearly blind and suffered from a heart condition. Sarah's mother was taking digitalis, a prescription drug that increased the force of her heartbeat. Because of her severe vision impairment, the medication was normally left out on the kitchen table where she could easily find it.

"I had left Sharelle in the living room playing, and had gone upstairs for a few minutes to get dressed," Sarah recalled. When she came back downstairs, she found her granddaughter in her mother's arms, being held over the kitchen sink and vomiting. "Mom, what happened" she asked in alarm.

"Sharelle's sick," her mother replied.

"I didn't know what the problem was at that time," said Sarah, who brought Sharelle back into the living room and had her lie down on the couch. "I thought it might be a touch of the flu coming on." When Sarah went back into the kitchen to get some water for Sharelle, she noticed for the first time that the top was off the container holding her mother's digitalis tablets, and that they were strewn across the counter. It was then that she realized that Sharelle must have swallowed some of the highly potent medicine. At that point, Sarah called her other daughter, Cheryl, who worked just down the street.

"My mother said, 'Sharelle has gotten into Gram's heart medication. She's vomiting. Come now.' My heart was pounding because I knew that Sharelle was a little girl and I knew that my grandmother's medication was rather serious because of her heart problems. When I got there, they didn't know how much medication she had taken. I started talking to her immediately, and kept trying to get her to tell me what exactly it was that she had done. She just kept repeating, 'I took my medicine.'" Sharelle was still vomiting and registering a very low pulse.

They decided it would be quickest to drive the 5 miles to the nearest hospital. "I realized that getting Sharelle to the nearest hospital was the most important thing," said Cheryl. They got the child to Windham Community Hospital within 10 minutes, and told the emergency-room staff that she had taken her great-grandmother's heart medication about 45 minutes earlier.

Herb Grey, the doctor in charge of the emergency room, described the situation: "The first thing we wanted to do was to get her on a cardiac monitor in order to determine if she had any apparent serious rhythm disturbance. The problem with digitalis is that it can have profound effects on the heart, including slowing of the heart or even cardiac arrest." By the time they got Sharelle on the monitor, the time-release medication was starting to take effect. Her heartbeat was slowly being suppressed. It was critical that they find out as soon as possible just how much of the drug had gotten into her system. "The blood tests that we did showed that she had indeed ingested digitalis and that her levels were four to five times above what would be considered toxic," said Dr. Grey.

In an attempt to lower the levels of the drug in Sharelle's system, she was given a special mixture of activated charcoal. "Activated charcoal is a specially treated charcoal that binds chemicals in the gastrointestinal tract and therefore prevents them from being absorbed into the bloodstream," Dr. Grey explained. Some of the mixture stayed in Sharelle's stomach for 3 or 4 minutes, but then she vomited most of it up, so it did not remain in her system long enough to have the desired effect.

Sharelle's condition continued to deteriorate. To her aunt's and her grandmother's increasing distress, she seemed to show no signs of improvement. "Watching the heart monitor and watching her blood pressure going up and down, I became more and more anxious, because I knew whatever it was that we were doing wasn't enough," said Cheryl. The decision was made to transfer Sharelle to Hartford Hospital's pediatric cardiology unit. "When they actually had her packaged up on the stretcher and the Lifestar door was open, and they put her into the helicopter and closed the door, I didn't think that I'd see her alive again," Cheryl said.

Sharelle's father, Ron, was contacted at work and told of her serious condition. "I don't know how I got from work to Hartford to see my daughter," he said. "I don't even remember half of the driving—I was just going. Too many things were going through my head. I just couldn't believe that this was actually happening. I thought I was going to wake up and discover that this was all just a bad dream. Lifestar was landing in the parking lot as I came in. I tried to get to the helicopter, but security wouldn't let me anywhere near it. I saw them take her out on a stretcher, and then it hit me that she was in really rough shape and in a fight for her life. I was yelling and screaming, calling for my daughter, just calling out, 'Sharelle, Daddy loves you. Please don't leave me.'"

Ron managed to get through to his wife, Pam, at another hospital, where she had just delivered a baby boy. "He told me that something had happened to our daughter, that she had taken Grandma's heart medication." Pam said. "That's when I asked him, 'Is she dead or alive?' And he said, 'Right now she's alive, but we don't know if she's going to make it or not.' At that point I thought that I had just given birth to one child, and that my other child was being taken away from me."

Cheryl went to the hospital to comfort Pam. "She looked up when I came through the door and she started to cry," Cheryl said. "I just went over to her and I held her and I said, 'Pam, she's going to be okay, she's going to be all right.' But none of us knew if she was or she wasn't."

Back at Hartford Hospital, the levels of the drug in Sharelle's bloodstream increased with each passing hour, but there was nothing more they could do. Unless the drug's levels became lethal, an antidote could itself be toxic. "I was just watching her with all that equipment—watching her heartbeat on the screen, praying that she wouldn't leave us, and wondering what I would do to myself for not having spent the time that I should have with my daughter," Ron said. Then, sometime later in the night, the levels of the drug in Sharelle's blood finally peaked, and it was clear that they would not need to use the antidote.

"It was about 2 in the morning when the nurse

came and told me that I could go in and see my daughter," Ron said. "They didn't have to tell me twice—I was gone. I stayed at her bedside with her for quite a while. Finally, she sat up, she took a drink of ginger ale for me, and we held each other for a while. She gave me a pretty big hug for a little kid."

Ron brought the good news to his wife, but it was 2 days before she was able to see her daughter. "She looked weak," Pam said. "And as soon as she saw me, she had a big smile on her face. She said, 'Mommy,' and put her arms out for a hug, and I went over and gave her a big hug, and cried."

Four years later, Sharelle had no permanent after-effects from the accidental overdose that nearly took her life. "Looking at her today, you wouldn't know that anything ever happened," Ron said. "She's healthy, active—you can't keep her down. She's just one bouncing beautiful girl."

"There are times when she may be sleeping in bed at night, and I just think back on the accident, and then I'll just go in bed and lie next to her and rub her, just feeling so thankful that she *is* with us today," Pam said.

"When the grandchildren come to visit, grandparents are not always aware of what may be of danger to children," Sarah said. "Not having children around, it's easy to forget that children are inquisitive and are going to touch things that they should not touch."

"Consider the fact that you have a lot of poisons that you normally use in your day-to-day activities," said Herb Grey, "mostly cleaning products that will be under the sink in your kitchen or under the sink in the bathroom, both areas that are readily accessible to a toddler, someone who's exploring their world."

"God didn't want her right now, and apparently she wasn't ready to go," said Pam. "To me, she is my miracle child. She has a long life ahead of her to live yet."

Signs and Symptoms of Poisoning by Ingestion:

➤ Nausea, vomiting, and diarrhea
➤ Severe abdominal pains and/or cramps
➤ Altered respiration and pulse rates
➤ Corroded, burned, or destroyed tissues of the mouth
➤ Unusual odors on the breath
➤ Stains around the mouth

Food poisoning represents a special case of poisoning by ingestion, and may cause some different signs and symptoms. The most common forms of food poisoning are bacterial. Suspect food poisoning if several people become ill with similar signs and symptoms at approximately the same time after eating the same food, or if one person becomes ill after eating food that no one else ate.

Botulism, probably the most serious kind of food poisoning, most often occurs after eating improperly home-canned foods. It is often fatal, and *always* constitutes a medical emergency.

Signs and Symptoms of Botulism (Usually Appear Within 12 to 36 Hours):

➤ Dizziness
➤ Headache

➤ Blurred and/or double vision
➤ Muscle weakness
➤ Difficulty in swallowing
➤ Difficulty in talking
➤ Difficulty in breathing

Medical attention should be sought immediately, preferably at the nearest hospital emergency department.

Mushroom poisoning occurs after eating certain wild mushrooms. Signs and symptoms appear within minutes to 24 hours, depending on the type and amount of mushrooms eaten, and may vary according to the type of mushroom.

Signs and Symptoms of Mushroom Poisoning (Any or All May Be Present):

➤ Abdominal pain
➤ Diarrhea (possibly containing blood)
➤ Vomiting (possibly containing blood)
➤ Difficulty in breathing
➤ Sweating
➤ Salivation
➤ Tears
➤ Dizziness

Salmonella poisoning usually occurs after eating fresh food that has been contaminated with salmonella bacteria. These most commonly include eggs, milk, raw meats, raw poultry, and raw fish. Salmonella poisoning can be very serious in infants, young children, the elderly, and the chronically ill. Signs and symptoms usually appear within 24 hours of eating the contaminated food.

Signs and Symptoms of Salmonella Poisoning (Any or All May Be Present):

➤ Abdominal cramps
➤ Diarrhea
➤ Fever
➤ Chills
➤ Headache
➤ Vomiting
➤ Weakness

Staphylococcus poisoning most often occurs from eating foods that have not been properly refrigerated. Most common among these are meats, poultry, eggs, milk, cream-filled bakery goods, and tuna and potato salad. Signs and symptoms usually appear 2 to 6 hours after contaminated food has been eaten.

Signs and Symptoms of Staphylococcus Poisoning (Any or All May Be Present):

➤ Abdominal cramps
➤ Nausea
➤ Vomiting
➤ Diarrhea

General Treatment for Poisoning by Ingestion:

1. Call a Poison Control Center and be prepared to give the following information:

- The victim's age
- Name of the poison (if known)
- How much poison was swallowed
- When the poison was swallowed
- Whether the victim has vomited. *Note:* if the victim has vomited and the poison is unknown, save some of the vomitus, which the hospital may analyze to identify the poison.

The Poison Control Center personnel will tell you what to do and if EMS personnel are required.

2. Do *not* administer the antidote listed on the label of the poison container unless advised to do so by a medical professional. The information provided by the manufacturer may be inaccurate, especially if the container is old.

3. Do *not* give the victim anything to eat or drink unless advised by a medical professional. If the poison has been ingested within the last 30 minutes, the Poison Control Center may advise you to dilute the substance by giving the victim milk or water to drink or to induce vomiting to empty the stomach and prevent absorption into the circulation system. *Never* give liquids to dilute the poison if the victim is unconscious or having convulsions. It is also generally inadvisable to give liquids to a person who has ingested poison in tablet or capsule form, since the increased fluid could dissolve tablets or capsules more rapidly in the stomach, speeding up the body's absorption of the poison.

Syrup of ipecac, available at your local pharmacy, can be used to induce vomiting. The normal dose for a person over 12 years of age is 2 tablespoons followed by two glasses of water. The dose for a person from 1 to 12 years of age is 1 tablespoon followed by two glasses of water. Vomiting usually occurs within 10 minutes. If this does not happen, repeat the dosage *only* once. If no syrup of ipecac is available, you can induce vomiting by tickling the back of the victim's throat with your finger or a spoon. Do *not* give mustard, table salt, or bicarbonate of soda (such as Alka-Seltzer) to the victim to induce vomiting.

Whether vomiting is induced or occurs spontaneously, steps should be taken to prevent the vomit from going into the victim's lungs or entering his trachea and choking him. Ideally, the victim should be seated and bent over, with his head lower than the rest of his body. If the victim is a small child, place him face down across your knees. Be certain to save a sample of the vomited material to bring to the hospital with you, or to give to EMS personnel if they are called to the scene.

Do *not* induce vomiting if:

- The victim is unconscious or semiconscious. In these states, he or she may inhale the vomit into the lungs.
- The victim is having a seizure.
- The victim has a serious heart problem.
- You do not know what the victim has swallowed.
- The poison is a strong *acid* or *alkali,* such as toilet-bowl cleaners, rust removers, chlorine

bleach, dishwasher detergents, or glucose-test tablets, or a *petroleum product,* such as kerosene, gasoline, furniture polish, charcoal lighter fluid, or paint thinner. Strong acids and alkalis are corrosive chemicals that damage or destroy tissues. Vomiting these corrosives could burn the esophagus, mouth, and throat. Petroleum products, if vomited, can be drawn into the lungs and cause a chemical pneumonia. The Poison Control Center will probably advise you to dilute these poisons with water, unless there are other, more dangerous substances combined with them in the product swallowed. In that case, they may tell you to induce vomiting to remove the greater risk.

4. If advised to take the victim to the hospital or to await the arrival of EMS personnel, keep the poison container and a sample of any vomited material available for examination and analysis. It is generally advisable to have all poisonings checked by a physician.

Treatment for Poisoning by Ingestion If the Victim is Unconscious or Having Convulsions:

1. Call EMS personnel.
2. Maintain an open airway (see p. 160) and restore breathing if necessary.
3. Loosen tight clothing around the victim's head and waist.
4. Do *not* give any fluids to the victim.
5. Do *not* induce vomiting. If the victim vomits on

his or her own, turn his or her head to the side so that the victim will not choke.

Tips for Preventing Poisoning by Ingestion:

- Become aware of the potentially toxic substances in your home (such as household cleaning products) and store them securely out of your child's reach. Almost 75% of all poisonings in children are due to household products.
- Securely store all household products in their original containers. Never store them in food or drink containers.
- Consider buying natural and nontoxic alternatives to your yard chemicals, pesticides, and sprays.
- Common toiletries are poisonous if ingested and should be stored out of the reach of children. These may include perfume, mouthwash, lotion, shampoo, and aftershave.
- Put Poison Control stickers (with the Poison Control hot line number) on all toxins in your home.
- Do not mix any medication with alcohol. The combination can be lethal.
- Don't share your medication. Prescription drugs should be taken only by the person for whom they were prescribed.
- Before administering an over-the-counter drug, read the warning label.
- Do not give or take medicine in the dark.
- Do not take or administer medication that is out of date, has no label, has begun to crumble, or has changed color or consistency.

- Dispose of small quantities of leftover medications by flushing them down the toilet rather than throwing them in the trash.
- Buy all medicine in childproof containers, but don't rely on them. Store them in a secured cabinet out of the reach of children.
- Always store medication in its original bottle. Do not put it in an unlabeled container or in a food or drink container.
- Do not keep vitamins on the kitchen counter. They present a poison hazard to children if ingested.
- Keep your purse out of the reach of children. It contains items that could be poisonous to them.
- Store liquor in a locked cabinet out of the reach of children.
- Look for a "nontoxic" label when buying crayons, paints, and other art supplies for your child.
- Post the phone number of your local Poison Control Center by your telephone, or put it into your automatic dialing system.
- To prevent food poisoning and the spread of bacteria, always wash your hands before and after handling raw meat, poultry, and fish.
- Cook meat, seafood, poultry, and eggs thoroughly to help prevent food poisoning. Avoid eating raw meat, seafood, and eggs.
- Never leave food standing. Bacteria thrive in lukewarm food. Keep hot foods hot and cold foods cold. Put leftovers away immediately.
- After handling your pet, wash your hands before handling food. Don't let your pet touch

food utensils or food surfaces. Pets are carriers of the same bacteria that cause food poisoning.

- Do not buy or use food if the expiration date has passed.
- Carefully examine all food containers for dented, rusted, swollen, or leaking seams. Do not open bulging cans.
- Become aware of which indoor plants are poisonous and present a hazard to children or pets. Mistletoe, poinsettias, and holly are extremely poisonous and should not be put in a house with children or pets.
- Do not eat unknown wild plants, berries, or mushrooms.
- During Halloween, check your children's treats before you allow them to eat anything they receive.
- Teach your children not to accept anything to eat, drink, or chew from a stranger.
- If you have severe food allergies of the kind that can lead to anaphylactic shock (see p. 10), learn the technical and scientific names for foods used in ingredient labels and always read the label before buying packaged foods.

CARBON MONOXIDE POISONING

Toxic or noxious fumes may stop respiration by a direct poisoning effect or by preventing the transport of oxygen by red blood cells. They can have an identifiable odor or be odor free. One example of a poison that can be inhaled in or around the home is carbon dioxide, which comes from decomposing organic matter, wells, and sewers. It is also in fumes from certain industrial and home spray chemicals.

Carbon monoxide, which is present in car exhaust fumes, is probably the most common of the poisonous gases, and is odorless, tasteless, and colorless. It can be produced by defective cooking equipment, defective heating equipment, fires, and charcoal grills, and is the result of incomplete combustion. Overexposure can be fatal. Carbon monoxide causes asphyxia (suffocation) because it combines with the hemoglobin of the blood much more readily than does oxygen. The blood therefore carries less and less oxygen to the body's tissues. The first signs and symptoms of asphyxia appear when a 30% blood saturation level has been reached.

The families of Randy and Johnna Chapman of Colorado Springs, Colorado, and of Tom and Ginny Lange of Roseville, Minnesota, both narrowly escaped death when this silent, invisible killer was unknowingly released into their homes.

In the fall of 1992, Randy and Johnna Chapman moved to Colorado Springs, full of excitement about their new home and Randy's new job. Just 6 days after the move, disaster struck.

"I work nights, so I had gone to bed earlier in the evening with my son, Brock. My wife and daughter were downstairs playing," Randy said, recounting the events of the evening. "All of a sudden, my wife discovered that my daughter wasn't feeling well."

"What's wrong with you?" Johnna asked 2-year-old Megan, who had suddenly lost all her enthusiasm for their game of catch. "Do you want to take a deep breath for Mommy, and see if you feel better?" Johnna said, holding her daughter in her arms. In response, the child simply closed her eyes and went limp. "Megan, Megan," Johnna called to her. "Megan, look at Mommy." There was no reply. "Randy!" the distraught mother screamed, instantly waking her husband.

Randy came downstairs and told his wife to call 9-1-1. Fire department dispatcher Marian Drucken-miller took the call.

"I have a little girl who's just turned 2," Johnna told her. "I was feeling her forehead and it felt like she had a temperature, like maybe she was coming down with something, like the flu. I gave her two children's Tylenol and she fell asleep. Now I can't wake her up!"

"Ma'am, we have help on the way," said Drucken-miller, reassuringly. "Is she still breathing?"

"Yes."

"The woman was real upset," Druckenmiller re-called. "She told me that her baby was convulsing and that she was real red. I thought that the baby had a high fever, and that she needed to cool her off." She repeated to Johnna that help was on the way, and told her that she needed to remain calm so she could help Megan. She instructed her to remove the child's clothes and to get a cool, damp rag and wipe her face.

"The whole time that we're doing these things to cool her off, she's still very lifeless, with no response," Randy said. "We had no idea what had happened, because she'd been healthy since the day she was born, and all of a sudden she's lying here lifeless in my arms, and I just wanted her back. I didn't want to lose her."

"I'm going to get hold of my paramedics who are responding to this call," Druckenmiller said. "They'll be there as soon as possible, but I want you to stay on the line while I talk to them." When Druckenmiller got back on the line to the Chapmans, Randy had taken his wife's place on the phone. "The paramedics are out in front of your house right now, so I'm going to let you go, and they're going to take real good care of her," she told the anguished father.

The Colorado Springs Fire Department had the first rescuers on the scene, including firefighter EMT Bud Whidmar, who rang the bell, knocked on the door, and called out to announce their arrival. "Nobody would answer the door," Whidmar said. "We couldn't hear anybody inside, and we kept beating on the door and calling out 'Fire department, fire department.' The longer we waited, the more we were getting concerned that something wasn't right. Then, just about when we were ready to force our entry, the father came to the door with the little girl in his arms. But he wasn't acting right. I asked him what was going on, but he didn't answer. It was as if he was in a stupor. I told my co-worker, Brian, 'This has all the signs and symptoms of carbon monoxide. Let's get them out of here, and get them out now.'"

Paramedic Brian Moffitt rushed Megan to the waiting medic unit. "Carbon monoxide is odorless, tasteless—it's not something you can detect. It's a very dangerous atmosphere," Moffitt said. "Really, your only treatment is to put the patients on a high flow of oxygen and take them to the hospital."

The EMTs began going through the house, looking

for victims and opening windows. "This was a very dangerous situation, because carbon monoxide kills within minutes," Whidmar said.

"Johnna," Randy called out, trying to locate his wife. He found her passed out in their bedroom upstairs. "Somebody, help!" he called.

"We told him to get out of the house three or four times, but he didn't want to do that," Whidmar said. "Then my concern went to the 7-year-old boy. I found him in his bedroom. I checked his breathing, and I couldn't find any breathing. Then I thought that we were really in trouble. When I picked him up, he started breathing on his own. I just grabbed him as fast as I could and ran out."

Firefighter EMT Dan Romero went to help Randy with his wife. "She was totally incoherent and her pulse was rapid," Romero said. "She was very, very close to death." Romero and Randy each took hold of one end of Johnna's body and started to carry her down the stairs and out of the house. About halfway down the staircase, Randy collapsed. "Help, I've got two people down here. Help!" Romero called. Three other EMTs rushed to his aid.

"A lot of people think that once you get out in the air that you can breathe okay," Whidmar said, "but the monoxide attaches itself to the blood cells. We have to force that carbon monoxide out and replace it with oxygen. We didn't have much time."

All of the victims, Johnna, Randy, Megan, and Brock, were taken to Memorial Hospital, where they were examined by emergency physician Michael Thompson. "The mother's level on arrival was 41, which means that that 41% of her hemoglobin was saturated with carbon monoxide," Thompson said. "I have actually seen patients die with levels less than 41. The father and son were essentially asymptomatic on arrival, even though they had significantly high carbon monoxide levels."

"The doctors explained to me that my wife had the most carbon monoxide in her system," Randy said, "so then my fears switched from my daughter to my wife, and I was very much afraid for her life."

"Due to the severity of poisoning of the mother and little Megan, we sent them to the hyperbaric oxygen chamber," Thompson said. "This is a chamber in which we can pressurize 100% oxygen to several atmospheres of pressure, and force carbon monoxide off the hemoglobin."

"My wife was lying inside the chamber with her eyes open," Randy said. "When she saw me, she touched the glass, and at that point I thought, 'She looks bad, but she's going to be fine.'"

While inside the hyperbaric chamber, Johnna and Megan were treated by Dr. Nathan Brightwell. "People should be aware that carbon monoxide poisoning, in its early stages, can seem very similar to flu-like illnesses," Brightwell said. "The Chapmans are very lucky in that Mrs. Chapman recognized that there was something wrong with her daughter Megan and called the paramedics."

"The mother and daughter were literally minutes away from death at the time that they were rescued by the paramedics, and the father and son would have followed shortly thereafter," said Thompson.

Johnna and her daughter were released from the hospital on the following day, without any lasting side effects. "You try to take every precaution possible to make sure that your family and your children are safe," Johnna said, "and to have something like this, which you cannot detect, come in and almost wipe your family out, is the scariest thing that ever happened to us. I cannot imagine what would have happened to us that night had we not had 9-1-1. I always knew how important it was, but now I know it's a lifesaver."

"When I see my kids and family today, sometimes I think of how, in a matter of seconds, one night it could all be taken away," Randy said. "But today, I'm just thankful that we're back to normal and my kids are full of life, just like they used to be."

It was discovered that the poisoning occurred because the Chapmans' furnace wasn't properly vented—a telling example of the fact that that home heating systems and fireplaces need to be inspected regularly. "We've had a fresh-air return put into the furnace room," Randy said. "We now keep the window open a crack, as we were told to do by the fire department, and we've purchased carbon monoxide monitors."

"It was really scary when I woke up in the ambulance, and I thought my sister was going to die," Brock said. "I would have missed having a little sister, because I love her more than anything."

A while after their brush with death, the Chapmans had the opportunity to talk with the EMTs who had saved their lives. "It was a real neat feeling to be able to hold the little girl, Megan, to be able to look at her and know that she was not going to suffer any ill effects from this, and that she was going to be able to go on to lead a fulfilled life," Bud Whidmar said.

"They acted so wonderfully and so professionally, and yet with such care," Johnna said. "They're just wonderful men, and we really appreciate what they did. What greater gift could anybody get than to have your family given back to you after coming so close to losing all of this?"

Early on the morning of November 7, 1991, Dr. Tom Lange and his wife, Ginny, were sleeping peacefully in their home in Roseville, Minnesota, when Tom was awakened by a loud thud. It seemed to come from the floor above them, where their eight children (seven of them adopted) were also in bed asleep. "I thought perhaps that this was one of our restless children who had fallen out of bed," said Tom. "But immediately after that, there was another thud and some crying, and I thought that I had to investigate that. When I reached the top of the steps, I saw Chuck lying face down in the bathroom."

"Chuck, what's wrong?" Tom asked his 10-year-old son, anxiously.

"I don't feel good," the child murmured in reply.

Twelve-year-old Dana was also collapsed on the floor. "Dana?" Tom said, baffled.

"I have a toothache," she muttered, groggily.

"Come on, you two, let's get going. Let me help you." Tom said, trying to lift Dana to her feet.

"I can't," Dana protested.

"Yes, you can walk," Tom insisted, pulling her into an upright position and guiding her out of the bathroom.

"Then I saw Tina in the hall, and asked her how she was doing, and she said she was sick, too," Tom said. "What I was thinking at that time was that several of the kids had the flu—and that wasn't unusual, to have three or four kids be sick in our household."

"A couple of kids are sick upstairs," Tom told his wife when he returned to their bedroom. "They've got the flu."

"I told Tom that I just couldn't get up then, because I just felt too nauseated," Ginny said.

"I'll take care of it," Tom replied. "I was trying to think through what could be going on—why would so many family members be sick?" Tom went to get some Tylenol, but when he went back upstairs he found another of his children, Jason, age 12, lying on the hallway floor, showing signs of a seizure. "It was at this point that I really became concerned," Tom said. He went to check on the rest of his children, and discovered to his dismay that they were all showing signs of sickness.

Suspecting that there might be a gas leak, Tom went down into the basement to check the heaters. "We hadn't been using our pool for about 2 months," he said, "but the burner seemed to be going full blast, and I couldn't turn it off. I didn't know what was going on, but I knew that heater shouldn't have been on like that. At this point, I felt a little woozy. As soon as I felt that myself, I became convinced that we were probably poisoned by carbon monoxide."

Tom opened several doors and windows throughout the house to let in fresh air, and then called the Poison Control Center. The dispatcher told him to get everyone out of the house quickly and over to the hospital. Tom and Ginny tried to round up all the children, but to no avail; they were all much too weak. In a panic, he called 9-1-1. The call came in to the Ramsey County Sheriff's Department. "This is Dr. Tom Lange," Tom told the dispatcher. "All of us woke up sick this morning. We're a family of 10."

"What do you think the problem is?" the dispatcher asked.

"I think it's carbon monoxide poisoning. I called the Poison Control Center."

"How sick is the sickest person there?" asked the dispatcher.

"We have coordination problems," Tom answered. "I have a van, but I don't think I can drive. I want to get my children down from upstairs."

"Can you keep them awake, and we'll send somebody right over?" the dispatcher asked.

"Okay," Tom said, and hung up the phone. Rescue units from the Roseville Fire Department were immediately dispatched.

"It was important to keep the kids moving and crawling and getting down to the fresh air," Ginny said, "because as long as they stayed where they were, they weren't going to be safe. They just wanted to lie down, and that's the only thing you want to do, because you're dizzy, you're nauseated, you're doubled up with pain in your stomach. The pain of this is excruciating."

"After my daddy called 9-1-1, I wondered if they were going to be there in time in order to save us," one of Tom and Ginny's daughters said. "All you're thinking at that moment is, 'Am I going to survive? Are we going to survive as a family?'"

Soon, the first rescue units arrived, including paramedic Denise Demars. "Carbon monoxide poisoning is real serious," Demars said. "And it's a cumulative thing—you can get more and more and more of it, and if you don't get rid of it, you can go into respiratory arrest, cardiac arrest, and you will die from it."

"The kids were so sick—we were so sick," Ginny

said. "You can't stand up; you can't move. Mobilizing those kids when they were that way—you hardly have the strength, but you know you've got to do it. It's like being in a fire—you've got to move. They kept saying, 'I can't, I can't,' and we kept saying, "You've got to, you've got to. This is your life.'"

Because of the large number of victims, extra rescue units from the Roseville Fire Department were dispatched. Within 10 minutes of the call, fire department rescue workers, including Fire Chief Joel Hewitt, began arriving at the scene. "I got out of the truck with my personnel and I told them to systematically search the house from the north end to the south end, looking in the bathrooms, in the closets, under the beds—wherever a person could be," Hewitt said. Outfitted with air packs, the firemen under his direction rushed into the house, gathered up the eight children and placed them in a large rescue vehicle, where Health One EMTs assessed their levels of carbon monoxide, administered 100% oxygen, and coordinated transportation to two different hospitals, one of which had a hyperbaric chamber to treat severe cases of carbon monoxide poisoning.

"They were all in different stages of consciousness," Hewitt said. "Some were vomiting, some had headaches. We had a steady stream of people coming down the stairs with victims in their arms."

"We knew we were in a race against time," paramedic Demars said. "We still had to get them to the hospital and we had to treat them. If carbon monoxide isn't cleared from the system, they could come out with permanent brain damage or permanent damage to the respiratory system or their hearts. The kids were not out of the woods, even though they were out of the house. My job was to try to assess all 10 people at once, and see who was the worst. I had them all look at me and I said, 'Raise your hand if you think you have to throw up. Now raise your hand if you have a headache. Now raise your hand if you have dizziness.' I knew that the person who raised his hand in response to all three questions was probably in a lot more trouble than the person who had two or only one of the signs and symptoms. Immediately, we routed those who were the sickest to the Hennepin County Medical Center, because they have a decompression chamber there. The people who were slightly less affected went first to Ramsey County Medical Center."

"I thought that all of us could have lost our lives within minutes—perhaps seconds. It was just too close," said Ginny later, although all 10 family members were treated and released without any sign of permanent injury.

Tom and Ginny were treated in the emergency room by Dr. John McGill. "Carbon monoxide poisoning is known as the silent killer," McGill said. "It's colorless, odorless, tasteless. And if it had occurred early in the night, they might have slept into unconsciousness and death, so I think they're all lucky to be alive."

An investigation showed that the heat exchanger on the pool furnace had corroded, causing dangerous gases to be blown back into the house.

"If you think that you are suffering from carbon monoxide poisoning, the absolute first thing to do is to get out of the area," said McGill. "The second is to call 9-1-1 or get to a hospital for evaluation."

A month after that near-fatal incident, the memories of that morning were still vivid for the whole large family. "My dad helped us through it all," one of the boys said. "If he hadn't gone down and checked on the furnace and realized what was going on, I probably would have died."

"We're definitely grateful to be alive, and we know that there were several elements of luck or fate that turned our way that morning," Tom said. "I've learned from this experience that we are very vulnerable to our environment, and I hope in some way that my family can be spokespeople about the silent killer that carbon monoxide is."

"The rescuers that were here that morning—I'm telling you, I was ready to hug every one of them," said Ginny. "They went right to work and did a superb job. I get goose pimples when I say that because they're great—they're fantastic."

"I think definitely the incident has brought us closer together as a family," said one of Tom and Ginny's daughters. "It's really, really scary to think that we all could have died that morning."

"The happiest moment was really seeing everybody okay," said one of their sons, "and I know that if we can get through that, we can get through anything."

Signs and Symptoms of Poisoning by Inhalation:

➤ Shortness of breath
➤ Coughing
➤ Cyanosis (bluish color)

Specific Signs and Symptoms of Carbon Monoxide Poisoning:

- ➤ Headache
- ➤ Dizziness
- ➤ Yawning
- ➤ Fainting
- ➤ Weakness
- ➤ Possible bluish color of lips and earlobes (not clearly visible in very dark skinned people)
- ➤ Possible bright red color all over body (not clearly visible in very dark skinned people)
- ➤ Nausea and/or vomiting

It is important to be extremely cautious when rescuing a victim from an area filled with poisonous gases or dangerous fumes, and, if possible, it is best to avoid attempting such a rescue alone. If you are outside the area of contamination, rapidly inhale and exhale two or three times, then take a deep breath and hold it before entering the area. At the site, attempt only to remove the victim or victims.

Treatment for Poisoning by Inhalation:

1. All victims of inhaled poisons need oxygen as soon as possible, so the first step is to get the victim to fresh air (upwind of poisonous fumes if they are outdoors) immediately.
2. Maintain an open airway (see p. 160). Restore breathing and circulation if necessary—rescue breathing (see p. 161) and CPR (see p. 229).
3. Loosen tight clothing around the victim's neck and waist.

4. Treat for shock (see p. 305).
5. Seek medical attention immediately, even if the victim seems partially or totally recovered, by calling 9-1-1 and informing the dispatcher of the need for oxygen, or driving to the nearest hospital emergency room.

Tips for Preventing Poisoning by Inhalation:

- Make sure you have adequate ventilation when using fuel-burning appliances. These appliances give off carbon monoxide gas.
- Never leave your car engine running in the garage. It is unsafe not only for someone in the garage but for anyone in the attached living space. Carbon monoxide can penetrate through any opening.
- When moving into a new house or apartment, have your gas heater checked by a professional before using it, to prevent carbon monoxide poisoning.
- Have your gas heater or furnace checked periodically to detect leaks.
- Learn how to shut off your gas appliance in case of a suspected leak or other emergency.
- Buy a carbon monoxide detector.
- If you think your gas stove is leaking, call the gas company, no matter what the time of day or night. Do not check by lighting a match, as you could cause an explosion.
- Be certain you have adequate ventilation when using products that give off fumes, such as paint, paint thinner, and varnish.
- Never mix household products. Many cleaners

contain either ammonia or bleach, which can let off a toxic gas when combined with other chemicals.

PLANT POISONING

Many poisonous substances in the form of gases, fumes, mists, liquids, oils, and dust can be absorbed by the body through the skin, irritating or poisoning the skin when they come in contact with it, and often affecting underlying tissues as well, especially hair follicles, oil glands, and sweat glands. Every year, millions of people suffer from contact with poisonous plants such as poison ivy, poison oak, and poison sumac. The poison comes mainly from their leaves, but may also leak out if you bruise their roots, stems, or berries. The smoke from burning brush containing these plants can carry their poisons a considerable distance. Contact with poisonous plants may result in any or all of the following signs and symptoms, some of which appear on the exposed skin surfaces 6 hours to several days after exposure.

Signs and Symptoms of Contact with Poisonous Plants:

➤ Redness of the skin
➤ Blisters
➤ Itching
➤ A red rash with some swelling, itching, and burning followed by formation of blisters of various sizes filled with blood serum. The blisters may fill with pus or contaminated fluid. When they break, scabs

and crusts are formed, and considerable fluid may be exuded.

➤ When the area affected is large and the inflammation is severe, there may be fever, headache, and overall body weakness.

Treatment for Contact with Poisonous Plants:

1. Immediately remove clothes close to or covering the affected area and wash the area thoroughly with soap and water.
2. Sponge with an oatmeal bath.
3. Calamine or similar lotions may be applied to prevent itching.
4. Antihistamines like Benadryl can be bought over the counter.
5. If the condition gets worse and large areas of the body or face are affected, the person should seek medical help to relieve the discomfort.

Other poisons commonly absorbed through the skin include dry and wet chemicals, such as those used in yard and garden maintenance, which may also burn the surface of the skin. After continued exposure to chemicals, inflammation may progress gradually. People who notice changes in the normal texture of their skin or continued irritation of the skin should seek medical advice before a chronic condition develops.

Treatment for Skin Contact with Dry or Wet Chemicals:

1. Call EMS system.
2. Remove contaminated clothing.

3. Flush the affected areas continuously with large amounts of water. If the contaminant is a dry chemical, such as lime, brush as much off as possible before flushing with water, being careful not to get any in your eyes or the eyes of the victim. Dry chemicals are activated by contact with water, but if continuous running water is available, it will flush the chemical from the skin before activating it. Continue flushing until EMS personnel arrive.

4. Monitor the person for signs of shock and changes in respiration.

To prevent poisoning by absorption, wear proper protective clothing for any activity that may put you in contact with a poisonous substance.

Seizure (Convulsion)

A seizure results from a disturbance in the electrical activity of the brain, which causes a loss of muscle control, sometimes manifesting as a series of uncontrollable muscle movements. These may occur during a state of total or partial unconsciousness, and there may be a loss of breathing.

Seizures can be the result of an acute or a chronic condition, the most common chronic condition being epilepsy, from which about 2,000,000 Americans suffer every year. Other causes include brain tumor, head injury, poisoning, electric shock, withdrawal from drugs, imbalances in blood sugar levels, heatstroke, scorpion bites, poisonous snake bites, hyperventilation, and high fever, particularly in infants and small children. They can range from mild blackouts that others may mistake for daydreaming to intense, uncontrolled muscular contractions (convulsions) lasting several minutes. Although seizures, especially of the convulsive kind, may appear alarming, they rarely cause serious problems in and of themselves. Injuries may result from falling during the seizure or from hitting against surrounding objects.

Signs and Symptoms of a Seizure (Any or All May Be Present):

➤ Before the seizure occurs, the victim may have a warning premonition or an aura. This is an unusual sensation such as a visual hallucination, a strange sound, taste, or smell, or the sense of an urgent need to get to safety.

➤ In mild cases, the victim may experience minor convulsive movements of the eyes or extremities.

➤ The victim utters a short cry or scream.

➤ The victim may become unconscious.

➤ Muscles become rigid, followed by jerky, twitching movements.

➤ There is a temporary cessation of breathing, or breathing becomes loud and labored, with a peculiar hissing sound.

➤ Just before the seizure, the face becomes pale, then turns bluish, especially in the lips, while the seizure is going on.

➤ The eyes may roll upward.

➤ There is a possible loss of bladder and bowel control.

➤ Drooling or foaming (possibly bloody) at the mouth may occur.

➤ Sometimes, severe spasms of the jaw muscles occur, causing the tongue to be bitten.

➤ The victim is unresponsive during the seizure, and may remain so for a period of time afterward.

➤ The victim may be sleepy and confused after the seizure is over.

It is important to remember that the person having a seizure cannot control the motions of his or her body, and that the object is to protect the victim from hurting himself or herself, not to try to stop the progress of the seizure.

1. If the victim starts to fall, try to catch him or her and lay him or her down gently. Protect the victim's head by placing a thin cushion, such as folded clothing, beneath it. If there is fluid, such as vomit, blood or saliva, in the person's mouth, position him or her on his or her side so that it can drain out.

2. Remove any nearby objects, such as furniture, which the victim might strike during the seizure, or remove him or her from dangerous surroundings, such as stairs, glass doors, windows, or a fireplace.

3. Do *not* hold or restrain the person in any way, or try to stop or control the muscular contractions. Holding or restraint can cause muscle tears or fractures.

4. Do *not* try to place any object, such as a spoon or a pencil, between the victim's teeth. Although people having seizures may bite their tongues or cheeks, they rarely do so with enough force to cause bleeding.

5. Do *not* throw any liquid on the victim's face or into his or her mouth.

6. Loosen tight clothing around the victim's neck and waist.

7. If breathing stops and does not start again momentarily after the seizure, maintain an open airway (see p. 160). Check to make sure the victim's tongue is not blocking his or her throat. Restore breathing if necessary.

8. Keep the victim calm and lying down after the seizure is over, since he or she may be drowsy, confused, or disoriented.

9. If the seizure has occurred in public, the victim may feel embarrassed or uncomfortable. Try to shield the victim from a crowd and keep curious bystanders at a distance.

10. Check for injuries, such as bleeding and broken bones, and provide appropriate treatment.

11. Seek medical attention. If the victim is known to have periodic seizures, it is not necessary to call EMS personnel. They should *always* be called if:

   • The seizure lasts more than a few minutes.
   • The victim has a second seizure.
   • The victim appears to be injured.
   • You are uncertain about the cause of the seizure.
   • The victim is pregnant.
   • The victim is a known diabetic.
   • The victim is an infant or child.
   • The seizure takes place in water.
   • The victim does not regain consciousness after the seizure.
   • The victim is HIV (human immunodeficiency virus) positive.

The most frequent cause of seizures in young children is a rapid rise in body temperature due to an acute infection. These are called febrile convulsions and usually occur in a child between 1 and 4 years of age. They seldom last more than 2 or 3 minutes.

The signs and symptoms are the same as for regular seizures.

Treatment for Seizures in Young Children:

1. Maintain an open airway (see p. 160). Check to make sure that the child's tongue is not blocking his or her throat. If it is, elevate the chin.
2. When the seizure is over, turn the child's head to one side or place the child on his or her side so that he or she will not choke if vomiting occurs.
3. Remove the child's clothing and sponge his or her body with tepid water to help reduce the fever.
4. Do *not* place the child in a tub of water, because he or she may inhale the water during the seizure.
5. Have someone call EMS personnel or the child's doctor during the seizure so that you do not leave him or her alone while it is happening. Otherwise, call when the convulsion is over.
6. Give Tylenol if the child is able to swallow. Do *not* give aspirin, as use of aspirin in children with a fever may lead to Reye syndrome.

Shock

Shock is the failure of the circulatory system to provide oxygen-rich arterial blood to all parts of the body. When vital organs are deprived of this blood, they stop functioning properly. This failure to function sets off a series of responses on the part of the body to try to maintain adequate blood flow to these organs. These responses result in a set of signs and symptoms that collectively are called shock.

The malfunctioning of the circulatory system that leads to shock can be caused by a large loss of blood, a dilation of the blood vessels beyond the capacity of the blood to fill them, or a weakness of the system's pump, the heart. These conditions can be precipitated by severe or extensive injuries; severe pain; severe burns; electrical shock; certain illnesses; allergic reactions; poisoning from inhaled, ingested, or injected toxic substances; exposures to extremes of heat or cold; emotional stress; or substance abuse.

The state of shock may develop quickly or may not take over until hours after the event that caused it. It occurs to some degree with every injury, and may be so slight that it is not noticed or so severe that it causes death, even when the injury itself would not normally prove fatal.

Signs and Symptoms of Shock (Any or All May Be Present):

➤ Restlessness or irritability (an early sign that the body is having a problem)

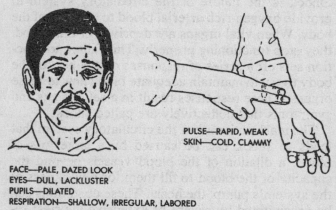

PULSE—RAPID, WEAK
SKIN—COLD, CLAMMY

FACE—PALE, DAZED LOOK
EYES—DULL, LACKLUSTER
PUPILS—DILATED
RESPIRATION—SHALLOW, IRREGULAR, LABORED

PERSON MAY BE PARTIALLY OR TOTALLY UNCONSCIOUS, DISORIENTED

Signs and Symptoms of Shock

➤ Dazed look (the result of reduced blood flow to the brain)
➤ Paleness in light-skinned individuals and ashiness or grayness in dark-skinned individuals (from blood being withdrawn from tissues near the surface of the body)

- ➤ Nausea and vomiting (believed to be caused by the involuntary nervous system losing control over certain small blood vessels in the abdominal cavity)
- ➤ Excessive thirst
- ➤ Weak, rapid pulse
- ➤ Cold, clammy skin (from reduced blood flow to extremities and nervous perspiration)
- ➤ Shallow, irregular breathing
- ➤ Dilated pupils
- ➤ Eyes dull and lackluster (from reduced blood supply)
- ➤ Weak and helpless feeling
- ➤ Anxiety
- ➤ Disorientation or confusion
- ➤ Unconsciousness (late stages of shock)
- ➤ Cyanosis (bluish color to skin, from extreme lack of oxygen—also late stages)

Instruction in first-aid emergency medicine, including treatment for shock, is often part of Boy Scout training programs. In the summer of 1993, 13-year-old Patrick Mizell, building a treehouse with some of his scouting friends, found out how important this can be.

Way up in a towering oak tree about 1 mile into the woods behind his house in Jackson, Mississippi, Patrick was working on the treehouse with his best friends, Ben Boteler and Pat Holloman, on the afternoon of August 28. They had constructed a ladder of planks nailed into the trunk of the tree, leading up to a high, broad branch, where they planned to construct the highest treehouse in the neighborhood.

Hearing the sounds of voices and hammering, two

other neighborhood boys, Maury Breazeale and Jonathan Daniel, joined them, and were appropriately awed by the scope and ambition of the project, which included bringing in building materials on a four-wheel off-road bike. "Those woods are kind of like my summer home," Maury said. "I'm back there a lot during the summer with my friends. We saw Patrick up in the tree, and he was about three or four stories high. I was amazed because I've never built a fort that high. We were talking about how awesome it was, and how cool it was going to be when it was finished."

The next thing they knew, someone up in the tree screamed, "Oh my God, Patrick!" as Patrick's body came hurtling down through the branches toward them. A small branch he had been standing on had unexpectedly given way.

"When Patrick hit the ground, it was one of the most terrible sounds I ever heard in my whole entire life," said Ben.

"He was lying on his side. He wasn't moving. And everybody was just running around screaming, 'What do we do? Oh my gosh, he's dead!' said Maury. "Ben and Patrick and I are all in the same Boy Scout troop, and when we earned the first-aid merit badge, they said that the worst thing you can do in an emergency is panic, because that's the way a lot of people die." Maury and Ben took charge of the situation.

"He's not breathing!" Ben shouted.

"I knew I was taking a chance because he might be paralyzed, but I had to turn him on his side to lift his chin up to open his airway," said Ben, who also checked to make certain that Patrick had a pulse. "Lifting his chin didn't work, so I did a finger sweep. His tongue was in the back of his throat, and I pulled it out."

"He's breathing, he's breathing," another of the boys called excitedly.

"His face was really pale," Maury said, "and in the Scouts there's a rhyme that says 'If the face is pale, lift the tail/If the face is red, lift the head.'" Maury told Ben to lift Patrick's legs so he wouldn't go into shock. The boys also took off their T-shirts and wrapped them around Patrick to help maintain his body temperature. "I was really scared for him," Maury said. "I wasn't sure if he was going to live or not."

Maury and Jonathan took the four-wheeler and went to the nearest house to get help. About 15 minutes after Patrick's fall, they got to a phone to call for EMS personnel. A mobile medical ambulance was immediately dispatched to the scene.

Back in the woods, Ben continued to hold Patrick's legs, encouraging and comforting him. "Hang in there, Patrick," he said. "You're going to be okay."

"Adrenaline was pumping through every vein in my body," Ben said, "and I really couldn't believe that this was happening. He was breathing very raggedly, and I thought he was going to die. Me and Patrick are great friends, and I just couldn't imagine him not being here anymore."

Paramedic Derrick Layton and the other rescue workers arrived at the nearest house within 25 minutes of the accident. "There was a lady waiting for us," Layton said. "She said, 'Get on the four-wheeler, and they'll take you to where the boy is.' The woods were about 100 yards back from the house, so I figured that we'd be right behind the house. But when we got there, we were probably a good mile away from where the ambulance was. I didn't have my radio with me because I didn't think I'd be that far out of contact with my crew. Just from looking at him, I knew that he was critical." Layton sent one of the boys back to his crew to get the equipment he needed.

Layton shouted, "Patrick, can you hear me?" and got no response. "I was surprised to see his blood pressure and his pulses as stabilized as they were," Layton said. "Everything that could have been done prior to our arrival was done. His eyes were gazed upward and to the right, which would indicate some kind of head injury. It crossed the back of my mind that he might die while we were still out in the woods."

Patrick's parents, Lori and Jim Mizell, were told of his accident and came racing through the woods to where he lay. "It seemed like I was running real fast," Lori said, "but I couldn't get there. It was like slow motion."

"I could tell by the looks on the faces of the paramedics and the firemen that it was a very serious situation," said Jim.

"Are you okay" Lori called to her son, distractedly.

"Ma'am, he'll be fine," Derrick Layton told her, reassuringly.

"He just looked to me like he was sleeping," said Lori. "I kept hoping against hope that he'd soon be okay. It's just that when you see your child sitting there, not moving, it's just kind of frightening."

"Since I lost my father, about 4 years ago, Patrick's been my biggest buddy," Jim said. "The thing that crossed my mind was that I was going to lose my best friend."

"It's real scary to think that you're going to outlive your child," Lori said. "I just would rather die than him die. He's such a joy—such a sweet, good kid."

Patrick, in critical condition, was taken to the trauma center at the University of Mississippi Medical Center, where he was treated by a team of doctors. "When I first saw Patrick, he was comatose," said Philip Azordegan, the neurosurgeon in charge of the case. He had sustained a punctured lung, but he hadn't broken either his neck or his back. The bad news was that he had sustained a very severe head injury. We were concerned that he either would remain in a coma permanently or would not survive at all."

Patrick's parents sat by his bedside, comforting him and trying to orient him to his surroundings. "Are you okay, sugar?" Lori asked.

"You okay, buddy? This is your daddy," said Jim. "You've got to go ahead and get well as soon as you can."

"We were just sitting there, trying to comfort him, telling him where he was, telling him what happened, so if he could hear us, he wouldn't be scared to death," said Lori.

"The main thing I was worried about was that his state of mind was going to get bad and he was just going to give up," said Jim.

"We got through that first night," Lori said, "and I kept telling him, 'This isn't good enough, Patrick. You've got to show me your eyes.' I just wanted him to wake up." Finally, Patrick raised his eyelids and looked at his thankful parents. "The first time I saw his eyes, it was like when you're looking at them when they're little babies, and they look at you and smile. He's just a bunch of prayers that were answered. He's just the answer to a prayer."

Patrick spent 10 days in the hospital, and proceeded to make an amazing recovery. "I think Patrick was an incredibly lucky young man," said his neurosurgeon. "I don't think anyone else who had fallen that distance would have done nearly as well or even survived that fall." Two months after he was released from the hospital, Patrick was back in school, begging to be allowed to go back to all his normal activities, including lifting weights.

"I'm learning to be real careful in trying the things that I do," Patrick said. "I'm learning that I'm not invincible."

"He's been very adventurous," Lori said. "Jim and I have said that if he makes it through his teens, it will be a miracle. We tease him now. We tell him that some angels caught him on the way down. It's probably what happened."

"The training that they had gotten in the Boy Scouts was the exact thing that he needed at that time," said Derrick Layton, the paramedic with the mobile ambulance crew that came to Patrick's aid. "If it hadn't been for them opening his airway, he would have been dead before we got there. There's just no question that they're the ones that saved his life."

"This accident has pulled us together," Maury said, "because we realize how fortunate we are that Patrick is here and that we all have such a good friendship. It really scared me to think that he was almost taken from us. I hope that nothing like that ever happens again. It was really hard."

"I don't think I can repay all the people that helped

me," Patrick said. "I want them to know that I'm very grateful for what they did."

"Maybe I'll get to see him grow up and see his kids," said Lori. "And when he has his own, he'll probably be able to feel the fullness of being a parent and the love that comes from it. He's my special son, and he always has been.

Though life threatening, shock is a reversible condition if recognized quickly and treated effectively.

Treatment for Shock:

1. **Call EMS personnel immediately.** A victim of shock requires advanced life support as soon as possible.
2. **Maintain an open airway** and ensure adequate breathing (see p. 160).
3. **Control bleeding** (see pp. 37–57).
4. **Keep the victim lying down,** if possible, and help him or her rest comfortably, in a position that will minimize pain. Intense pain can increase the body's stress and accelerate the progression of shock. Make sure that the head is not lower than the body. Handle the victim gently, and minimize movement.
5. **Elevate the legs** to keep blood circulating to the vital organs, if the injury will not be aggravated by this (there are no broken bones in the hips or legs) and there are no head or abdominal injuries. If the victim is suffering from head injury, sunstroke, heart attack, stroke, or shortness of breath due to chest or throat injury, it may be necessary to raise the head and shoul-

ders. With head injuries, however, there is a high probability of spinal damage, and if there is any question of this, it is best to keep the victim flat.

6. Loosen any tight clothing constricting the neck, chest, and waist to facilitate breathing and circulation.

7. Provide the victim with plenty of fresh air.

8. Unless the victim is suffering from heatstroke, help the victim maintain normal body temperature by wrapping in blankets, clothing, or other available material. These coverings should be placed under the victim as well to minimize the loss of body heat.

9. Do not give the victim anything to eat or drink. Surgery may be required and is best performed when the stomach is empty.

10. Calm and reassure the victim. Do not discuss his or her injuries or allow others to do so in his or her presence.

Sprains and Strains

Sprains and strains are injuries that occur to muscles, tendons, and ligaments. They are usually quite painful, though rarely life threatening. If not quickly taken care of, however, they can become permanently disabling. It is important therefore to identify them and treat them properly.

Rest, ice, and *elevation* are the general first-aid treatments for all sprains and strains. The application of ice or cold compresses causes the blood vessels at the injury site to constrict, limiting the amount of blood and other fluid that seeps out, thus reducing the swelling. It also reduces muscle spasms and numbs nerve endings, thus helping to limit the pain. Elevation of the injury above the level of the heart reduces swelling in the area.

Heat may be applied after a period of time designated by a physician, if the swelling has gone away. This will speed up the healing process by dilating the blood vessels and allowing white blood cells and other cells that help repair tissue to move more quickly into the injured area. *Never* apply heat immediately after an injury or while the area is still swollen.

If the injury is serious, it may have to be immobilized before ice is applied or the area is elevated. The purposes of immobilization are to reduce pain, prevent additional damage to soft tissues, limit the risk of serious bleeding, and prevent loss of circulation to the injured part. If you decide to transport the victim to a medical facility, it is wise to immobilize the injured area before moving him or her.

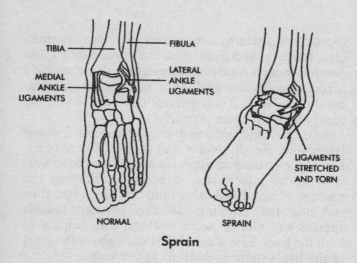

TIBIA

FIBULA

MEDIAL ANKLE LIGAMENTS

LATERAL ANKLE LIGAMENTS

LIGAMENTS STRETCHED AND TORN

NORMAL

SPRAIN

Sprain

A *sprain* is a stretching or tearing of the ligaments or other tissues at a joint. It is usually caused by a sudden twist or overextension of a joint, forcing the bones farther apart than the normal range of motion of the joint permits. The most commonly sprained joints are those of the wrist, fingers, ankle, and knee.

A mild sprain is one in which the ligaments are only stretched or a few of their fibers are torn.

These generally heal rapidly, causing pain and discomfort for only a few hours. If they are not treated and not properly rested, however, the joint is often reinjured. Unlike fractures, which usually heal leaving the bone as strong as it was before, the stretched or torn ligaments of a sprained joint usually do not regenerate, and if not surgically repaired, make the area subject to repeated injury.

A severe sprain, in which a number of ligaments are torn, may require weeks of medical care before normal use is restored to the joint. In a severe sprain, the bones may also become dislocated or even broken. The stretched ligaments may pull the bone away from its point of attachment to the other bone or bones in the joint.

Signs and Symptoms of a Sprain:

> Pain on movement of the injured area
> Swelling at the joint
> Tenderness to the touch
> Discoloration (black and blue) of the skin around the injury

It is sometimes difficult to distinguish between a sprain and a closed fracture. If in doubt, treat the injury as if it were a fracture (see p. 127). The general principles of rest, ice, and elevation can be applied, followed by heat after the swelling has disappeared.

Treatment for Sprains of the Ankle or Knee:

1. Elevate the area of the sprain above the level of the heart, if possible, in a position of complete

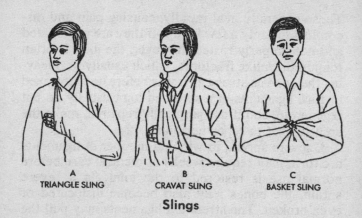

| A | B | C |
| TRIANGLE SLING | CRAVAT SLING | BASKET SLING |

Slings

rest. This will help slow the flow of blood to the injury site and reduce swelling.

2. Apply an ice bag, a cold compress, or a chemical cold pack to the area intermittently for the first 12 or 24 hours to reduce swelling and relieve pain. Do *not* apply ice directly to the skin.

3. Seek medical help if swelling or pain persists.

Treatment for Sprains of the Shoulder, Elbow, or Wrist:

1. Place the injured arm in a sling. A sling is a support made from a triangular bandage. To make a triangular bandage, cut a piece of cloth 36 to 40 inches square, and then cut the square in half along the diagonal. To make a sling from the bandage:

   a. Place one end of the base of the triangle over the shoulder of the uninjured side, allowing

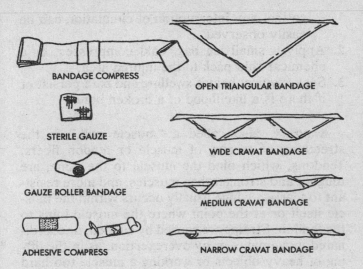

BANDAGE COMPRESS

OPEN TRIANGULAR BANDAGE

STERILE GAUZE

WIDE CRAVAT BANDAGE

GAUZE ROLLER BANDAGE

MEDIUM CRAVAT BANDAGE

ADHESIVE COMPRESS

NARROW CRAVAT BANDAGE

Dressings and Bandages

the rest of the bandage to hang down over the chest, so that the apex of the triangle lies behind the elbow of the injured arm.

b. Bend the injured arm at the elbow, across the chest, on top of the bandage, so that the hand is elevated 4 to 5 inches above the elbow.

c. Bring the lower end of the bandage up over the injured arm to the shoulder of the uninjured arm, and tie it to the other end there, making certain the knot is at the side of the neck.

d. Fold the apex of the triangle and pin it to the outside of the bandage, or twist it and tuck it in at the elbow.

e. Make certain that the fingertips are exposed,

so that any interruption of circulation can be easily observed.

2. Apply a small ice bag, cold compresses, or a chemical cold pack to the injured area.

3. Seek medical help if swelling and pain persist or if there is a likelihood of a broken bone.

A *strain,* also called a "muscle pull," is the stretching or tearing of muscle or tendon fibers. Tendons, which bind the muscle to the bone, are tougher and stronger than muscles, and more resistant to tearing, which usually occurs within the muscle itself or at the point where the muscle joins to the tendon. Strains are caused by sudden, uncoordinated movements or by overexertion, as in the lifting of heavy objects or working a muscle too hard or too long. The muscle areas most commonly strained are the neck, the back, the thigh, and the back of the lower leg. Strains are often neglected, which can lead to reinjury of the strained area.

Signs and Symptoms of a Strain:

➤ Intense pain
➤ Moderate swelling
➤ Increased pain and discomfort with movement
➤ Sometimes, discoloration

Treatment for a Strain:

1. Rest the affected area immediately, putting the victim in a comfortable position.

2. If possible, elevate the injured area.

3. Apply an ice bag or other source of cold to the area to reduce swelling.
4. After 48 hours, apply warm, wet compresses to the area.
5. If pain or swelling is persistent or severe, seek medical attention.

For tips for preventing sprains and strains, see Tips for Preventing Dislocations and Fractures, p. 151.

Stroke

A stroke, also called a cerebrovascular accident, occurs when the blood supply to part or all of the brain is interrupted to a degree that causes damage to brain tissue. It can be caused by a blockage or constriction of an artery carrying blood to the brain. The most common cause is a clot (called a thrombus or an embolism) that forms or lodges in one of the arteries that supplies blood to the brain. High blood pressure or fat deposits lining an artery (atherosclerosis) may also cause stroke. More infrequently, it may be caused by a tumor or swelling from a head injury that compresses an artery. The effects of a stroke on the brain can be temporary or permanent and range from slight to severe.

Signs and Symptoms of a Stroke (Any or All May Be Present):

➤ Victim looks ill or begins behaving abnormally
➤ Sudden headache
➤ Sudden paralysis, weakness, or numbness of face, arm, or leg on one side of the body; a corner of the mouth may droop

- ➤ Decreased level of consciousness or complete unconsciousness
- ➤ Slurred speech or inability to speak
- ➤ Mental confusion, including inability to understand speech
- ➤ Sudden fall
- ➤ Impaired vision (dimmed or blurred)
- ➤ Pupils of the eyes are of two different sizes
- ➤ Respiration is slow, with a snoring sound caused by the tongue falling back into the airway.
- ➤ Difficulty with breathing, chewing, and/or swallowing
- ➤ Dizziness
- ➤ Changes in mood
- ➤ Ringing in the ears
- ➤ Loss of bladder and/or bowel control
- ➤ Strong, slow pulse

Treatment for Stroke:

1. Call EMS personnel. Consider the possibility of a head or spinal injury, and if it appears to be present, modify first-aid procedures accordingly.
2. If the victim is unconscious, maintain an open airway (see p. 160). If there is fluid or vomitus in the mouth, position the victim on his or her side to allow it to drain out. You may have to do a finger sweep to remove some of the material.
3. Restore the breathing if necessary (see p. 161).
4. Keep the tongue or saliva from blocking the air passage.
5. Keep the victim lying down, with his or her head and shoulders raised to alleviate some of the pressure on the brain. If the victim is uncon-

scious, place the victim on the affected side to allow fluids to continue to drain. Do not move the victim more than is necessary.

6. Do not give the victim anything to eat or drink.
7. Keep the victim quiet and calm.
8. Reassure the victim, who may become extremely anxious or not understand what has happened to him or her.

Transient ischemic attack is a temporary episode caused by a spasm of a cerebral blood vessel, and is sometimes called a "ministroke." Like a stroke, it is caused by reduced blood flow to part of the brain, but its signs and symptoms disappear within a few minutes or hours. It usually occurs in individuals between the ages of 50 and 70. Despite its transience, the victim is not necessarily out of danger once the signs and symptoms pass. A person who experiences a transient ischemic attack is 10 times more likely to have a stroke in the future than one who does not.

Signs and Symptoms of a Transient Ischemic Attack (Any or All May be Present):

➤ Slight mental confusion
➤ Slight dizziness
➤ Minor speech difficulties
➤ Muscle weakness

Since the signs and symptoms cannot be clearly distinguished from those of stroke, it is best to seek professional medical attention immediately for treatment for further evaluation.

Index

319